A Journey
of Faith

A Journey of Faith

A Mother's Alzheimer's, a Son's Love, and His Search for Answers

Edward Grinnan

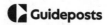

A Journey of Faith

Published by Guideposts Books & Inspirational Media,
100 Reserve Road, Suite E200, Danbury, CT 06810
Guideposts.org

Scripture quotations marked (NKJV) are taken from *The Holy Bible, New King James Version*. Copyright © 1982 by Thomas Nelson.

Cover and interior design by Pam Walker,
W Design Studio LLC
Cover photo by Amy Etra Photography
Typeset by Aptara, Inc.

ISBN 978-1-959634-90-4 (hardcover)
ISBN 978-1-961125-07-0 (epub)

Printed and bound in the United States of America
10 9 8 7 6 5 4 3 2 1

For my family

The heart that has truly loved never forgets.

—THOMAS MOORE

Contents

Introduction

I peered out the kitchen window into the moonless winter night, the fresh snow blanketing our yard barely a shadow, and wondered, *Did I remember?*

"Can you see her?" I called upstairs to Julee.

"No."

Julee's vantage point was superior to mine. She was better able to track our golden retriever Gracie's movements, thanks to the bright green collar light I always turn on before letting her out at night up here in the Berkshire Mountains of Western Massachusetts. But had I? Had I remembered? I *always* remembered, until recently, it seemed.

"Maybe the battery is dead," Julee said. No, I'd just replaced that collar light. At least I remembered to do that.

A sickening panic stirred within me. Not out of fear for Gracie. She could handle herself at a lean, fearless seventy-five pounds. Besides, the bears were all asleep for the winter. No, this was fear for myself.

There is a strong history of Alzheimer's dementia in my family. My mother died of it, as did both her sisters, one of her brothers who may have fallen victim before a stroke killed him, and my Pop-Pop, the only grandparent alive in my lifetime. My memories of him are fuzzy and I was too young to understand why he had such trouble remembering my name or whom I belonged to. That memory deficit came in handy, though, when he couldn't recall if he had given me the customary quarter he always bestowed when I visited and slipped me another one, and sometimes a third. "Did I give you your quarter yet?" he'd ask, and I'd shake my head in mock shyness, thinking it was all a game.

Among the current generation some of my older cousins on my mother's side are already showing possible signs. Maybe that's why I have developed this near phobic reaction to even the most minor misfire of memory. The slightest lapse can set off an inner frenzy of doubt about my own brain health and start me brooding about my family's history and my own susceptibility. It feels at times as if I am trying to outrun my own shadow.

"There she is!" Julee shouted. "Down by the apple tree."

A minute later, a cheerful bark at the side door proclaimed that Gracie was ready to be let back in and receive her bedtime treat. Removing her collar, I noticed that the light was indeed off. Julee guessed that Gracie might have extinguished it herself, rolling in the snow, which she enjoys, crazy golden that she is. I wasn't so sure.

My mother was diagnosed with Alzheimer's about thirty years ago and died eight years later, several years after her older sisters, Marion and Cass, both died in memory care units. This book, in part, tries to sketch out that journey and the impact the disease has had on her children, who ultimately became her caregivers: my brother Joe, a lawyer; my sister Mary Lou, a school psychologist; and my sister-in-law, Toni, also a lawyer and the most practical person I've ever known. Then there was me, the youngest who everyone said was Mom's favorite, living in New York, which sometimes felt like light-years away from Michigan, where Mom and my siblings, who took on so much responsibility for her care, all lived.

The Alzheimer's journey is a difficult one millions of families have traveled, filled with pain and anger, empathy and hope, faith and prayer, and even on occasion joy. Ours was no different, as you will learn.

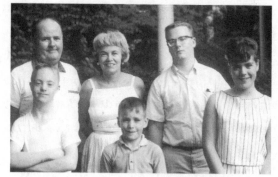

My family in 1962. Back row: Dad, Mom, and Joe.
Front row: Bobby, me, and Mary Lou.

Yet looking at my family only makes me look at myself, at my own complicated relationship with the specter of Alzheimer's. Watching my mother slip inescapably into dementia, like a schooner slowly disappearing into a fogbank, its sails billowing with an implacable wind, compels me to dwell on my own vulnerability. I understand one's genetics are a fifty-fifty proposition. Although my father died in his early seventies of heart disease a few years before my mother showed symptoms of dementia, I take so much after my mom, from her grass-green eyes to her eruptive giggle. "You're just like her," I've always heard. The resemblance is unmistakable.

So is the bunion on my right foot whose pain level rises and falls with the barometer. Only recently did I understand why Mom would moan, "My toe is killing me." What else might I have inherited from her? And if there is a ticking bomb concealed in my brain matter, do I want to know?

Wanting to know is the key. Knowing is one thing—you can know something without wanting to know it. *Wanting* to know is quite another. Wanting to know is what makes us human. Wanting to know the future, wanting to know love, wanting to know ourselves, wanting to know and love God. If there is a way to predict that I, too, will slip into that miasma, do I want to know it? Accept it? Prepare for it? Deny it? Dread it?

I hope to answer these questions in the pages that follow, as well as let you hear from other families and individuals who have known the struggle of Alzheimer's, especially those who have told their stories in *Guideposts* magazine, of which I am the editor-in-chief, and at Guideposts.org, where I publish a weekly blog about this journey and invite your contributions. It is especially those responses that have inspired and motivated me, like this one from Mary G.

"I'm there with you, Mr. Grinnan. My sister passed away with Alzheimer's and my mom passed away with it in 2003. To see what that awful disease can do to a person is frightening. For quite a while I let the fear run my life and beat myself up when I would forget any little thing. But with a lot of prayer and God's great mercy I am doing much better and trying to enjoy each and every day to the fullest. I'm not letting the fear take over my life. And I keep telling myself it may never happen anyway. Take care and be happy!"

I have become convinced we are a country collectively and individually trying to come to grips with a disease that steals our memories, our very ability to think. If the great French philosopher and mathematician René Descartes was correct—we think, therefore we are—Alzheimer's deprives us of the very faculty that makes us a person, that defines our existence. What other disease does that to the ones we love? To ourselves? What other disease erases who we are?

The night of what I've come to call the "collar light incident" I lay in bed staring sleeplessly at the ceiling, pondering the state of the 86 billion neurons—give or take—thrumming inside my skull. I couldn't dispel one researcher's words I read describing the disease's preclinical stage: "By the time [early] symptoms appear, protein build up has already damaged the brain neurons. The plaque is destroying the neurons' ability to serve as a giant communications network to allow different parts of the brain to communicate with each other and to internal organs and other body parts. Until we find a cure, from the time Alzheimer's begins, it is a slow march to the grave."[1]

No wonder I couldn't sleep. Even an owl's gentle onomatopoeic hooting didn't soothe me. Fear was winning and I couldn't let that happen. Yet nothing could be more frightening than something brewing undetected in your brain that will ineluctably strip away everything

---

[1]*Dementia Types, Symptoms & Risk Factors, p.265, The Jerry Beller Health Research Institute*

that makes you you, and knowing there is nothing you can do about it. You don't even know it's happening until it's too late.

I thought back to the signposts of my mother's illness. When did it start? What did we miss? Is there a moment when you know or is it an accretion of incidents? It's hard to say.

I remembered visiting her once back in Michigan with Julee. Mom was making coffee for our breakfast. She was a whiz at cooking bacon and eggs and toast and timing it all perfectly. But suddenly Julee shouted. Mom had forgotten to put the carafe under the drip basket and coffee was overflowing all over the place. Mom couldn't remember what she'd done with the carafe, but

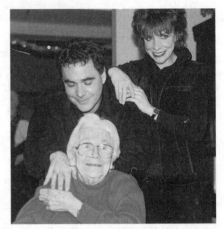

Mom, me, and Julee in 1998.

I finally found it in a cabinet and got it in place while Julee sopped up the mess. Mom seemed strangely indifferent to the whole episode and Julee reminded me that Mom usually had tea in the morning. We didn't mention it again, and I hadn't even thought about it until now.

Not very long ago I'd done the exact same thing with our single-cup coffee maker. I'd put the pod in place and dutifully started the brewing process only to hear Julee yell seconds later, "You forgot the cup!" Admittedly it was Monday morning, but it was to be my second cup of coffee and I had no excuse. And as I tossed and turned, I tried not to recognize the similarities between my slip of memory and my mother's and having to sop up the mess with paper towels. It had been the start of a busy week. I'd stayed up too late the night before. I had a lot on my mind. Yet still…

The next day I unburdened myself to an old friend. I told him how every little slip of mind, every time I found myself confused when I shouldn't be, eroded my faith in my ability to think, to someday be able to even function.

"I'm convinced these incidents are becoming more frequent," I said. "I'm keeping track. I want to know what they mean."

My friend stared at me for a long time. Then he exploded in laughter.

"You want to know what they mean? Are you kidding me?" he said. "If I stressed out every time I forgot something, which I do all the time, I definitely couldn't function. Dude, we forget more stuff than we ever remember in life, trust me. Lighten up. Remember, we put our lives in the hands of a loving God. We are not in this alone. If your faith can't help you with this, I don't know what can. *There's your answer.*"

He was making a reference to the language of AA, where we'd met years before when he was just trying to get clean and I was finally finding my feet in sobriety after years of struggle. Some days it felt like I was still finding my feet. Today, after more than twenty-five years without a drink, I worry that years of alcohol and drug abuse increase my chances of brain decline. Alcohol in particular can cause dementia—wet brain, it's called—all on its own. How wet was my brain before I eventually dried out? I'd had neurological symptoms during my many withdrawals—convulsions, hallucinations, panic attacks. I suffered several concussions during my drinking years, and perhaps a few more I

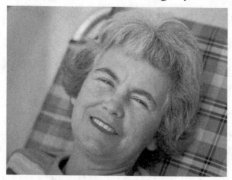

Mom, circa 1960.

wasn't even aware of. I wanted to know if these insults to my brain matter increase my susceptibility to dementia.

By comparison, my mother was very healthy. She never smoked, was a light alcohol user (I never saw her even tipsy), and certainly didn't use drugs. She wouldn't even take an aspirin. She exercised, played point guard for her college basketball team even. And yet she succumbed to a fatal dementia that seemed practically inescapable in her family.

"We can't control what we can't control," my friend added, quoting one of the program's popular slogans, which he knew I hated.

Finally, I cracked a smile. "I know," I said, "a day at a time. Keep it simple. Live in the now. Let go and let God."

And still, I couldn't help thinking—isn't that what Alzheimer's does in its own insidious way? Traps you in the now. Shrinks the aperture of our perceptions until all we know is what we know at that moment, life reduced to a confusing pinhole in time. I thought of my mother toward the end. The past was the present, the present the past. Her mind was a house of cracked mirrors.

I'm fairly sure that writing this book won't answer all my questions or quell my angst. I plan to undergo neurological testing and whatever else that can predict or even diagnose Alzheimer's. I've already done a number of cognitive tests, albeit online, inevitably followed by a barrage of ads for potions and supplements and elixirs guaranteed to restore my mind, even improve it. The results of some of these tests were clearly suspect. I don't think I could have passed them even in graduate school. But they made me a mark for marketers. Others, though, seemed more legit, and some of the results had me worried.

I've embarked on this journey with open eyes and heart. I've prayed about it without being sure I got an answer, which might itself be an answer. God's silence challenges us to draw on our own inner resources. Or maybe He just thinks I'm crazy.

It is the wanting that pulls me, the wanting to know, that primal yearning. It's not how everyone feels. I would say from the responses to my blog it's about fifty-fifty. Some people want to prepare themselves and their families. Some want to arrange caregiving and finances. Some want to enroll in experimental treatment programs. Most say they will lean into their faith—hard. Others simply don't want to know and are afraid to even think about it. I can't blame them.

Some, like me, just want to know because knowing is better than not knowing, as a matter of principle. Knowledge is armor. And if I find that answer, elusive as it may be, I plan to share it with you.

In the meantime, I will defer to the advice of Mary G: I will take care and be happy…and try not to spill the coffee all over the place.

• • •

CHAPTER ONE

WHAT MAKES US HUMAN

There is so much I want to tell you about my mother that no book I could write would have enough room for everything I want to say.

She was smart, the daughter of a schoolteacher who taught her to read before she even started school, and skipped several grades. She was opinionated to a fault, some might say, maybe because she read several newspapers a day, to say nothing of the book or two she was always in the middle of. She was a TV game show winner back in the '50s. She was devoted to her church and to her faith (lots of opinions there, too, often to my conservative father's consternation), and the mother of a son with Down syndrome. She volunteered for everything, including being the den mother of my brother Bobby's Cub Scout troop for kids with Down.

In truth my mother could be a little absent-minded, but we always wrote that off to the many activities she was involved in. My father called her scatterbrained, but I believe that was because he was so rigidly organized; he always showed up way early for church so we could sit in the exact same pew we always did. Mom was a competent but indifferent housekeeper—same with cooking—because there were more important things in life. So, when little shortcomings emerged, like the coffee episode, or she left a burner on the stove on overnight, we wrote it off. Or at least I tried to. *That's just Mom,* I told myself when I heard about these things.

Some of Mom's earliest problems showed up at church, not surprisingly. Mom spent a good deal of her life at St. Owen's, especially after my father's death. One of her duties was to count the collection basket every weekday after morning Mass, fill out a deposit slip, and take it to the bank. Several days a week she manned the desk at the church library and was responsible for, among other things, shelving books. She would also help our pastor, Father Walling, with paperwork and the weekly bulletin, and was part of the altar society. Church kept her busy. It was her refuge.

It was Sister Carolyn, her favorite nun and a friend in recent years, who alerted us to Mom's growing problems at St. Owen's.

"She's a bit confused when counting the basket," Sister told Mary Lou. "The teller at the bank usually catches it and makes out a new deposit slip. So, from now on I'll quietly recount the basket before we go to the bank. I don't want to embarrass your mother. I know how important this is to her. She wants to be of service, and we can't take that away from her."

"Father Walling has also noticed that she's having some difficulty with her librarian duties," Sister continued. "Some of the books she shelves have to be reshelved correctly. So, we might tell her she needn't do that anymore, though of course we'll keep her at the desk welcoming people and checking books in and out. Again, we don't want to upset her. You know how proud she is. She needs to feel needed."

That was exactly right. Mom did need to feel needed. She was lost without having something to do and someone to do it for. Away from her church obligations she worked at The Resource Center, helping distribute used furniture to families in need. My dad called her a liberal do-gooder; I doubt he meant it as a compliment, but she took it as one.

Sister Carolyn's concerns—she called them "signs"—were worrying to some degree. But who couldn't say it was just the minor failings of an aging brain? I can't fill out a bank deposit slip without using the calculator on my phone and even then the teller sometimes has to redo it. I've resorted to simply making deposits digitally.

Sister Carolyn was both Mom's friend and confidant. Mom was educated by nuns, as I partly was, and had great reverence for them.

I'm sure she told Sister Carolyn things she told no one else, which told me those signs Sister was noticing might be more than minor slips.

Signs. Even though her dad and both of her sisters had Alzheimer's, the disease was not necessarily considered inheritable, especially not thirty years ago. The odds were in her favor, were they not? It couldn't strike all four of them. I tried not to imagine her counting and recounting the collection basket and how hard she must have tried to suppress the apprehension that she surely must have felt when the amounts never came out the same. She was good at math. It absolutely broke my heart to think about it, so I didn't.

Yet it was that word—*Alzheimer's*—that seemed to have a power all its own. No one wanted to say it, least of all me. I loved my mom, but I hated that word. It's as if the two could never coexist in my mind.

• • •

ALZHEIMER'S WAS A DISEASE OF THE MIND LONG before it bore the name of German physician Alois Alzheimer, who first described its symptoms and progression in 1906. His descriptions were based on a female patient he identified only as Auguste D., whom he had begun seeing in 1901 until her death five years later.

Before that we used many terms to describe the erosion of mental faculties with the onset of old age. Senility was the most prominent, derived from the Latin *senex*, meaning old, old man, and later from the French *senile*, meaning of old age or dotage. Since a word or term exists in most cultures describing age-related memory loss and cognitive decline, pathological or otherwise, we can assume that dementia has been with us for as long as we have been human.

Indeed, many species of primates, as well as dogs, cats, and other mammals, are documented as being similarly afflicted. The fact that humans live longer than ever in much of the world has increased the diagnosis of age-related brain disease. In fact, classical Alzheimer's originally applied only to what we now call early-onset Alzheimer's. It wasn't until the 1990s that the diagnosis was modified to include geriatric patients.

It was Shakespeare, of course, who drew the most vivid literary picture of dementia unleashed in his great tragedy, *King Lear*. The eighty-year-old Lear is a man whose mind is clearly in a horrifying tailspin. His decisions become increasingly delusional and destructive until, in his abject confusion, he cries out, "Who is it that can tell me who I am?" In fact, a few neurologists have speculated that Lear suffered from Lewy body dementia, a particularly aggressive form of dementia that intersects with Parkinson's. I believe Shakespeare was aggregating all he had observed in human aging in one epic figure, for there was no greater observer of human behavior than the Bard.

There have been many notable and famous people who have succumbed to Alzheimer's and related dementias. The list includes Pat Summitt, Norman Rockwell, Gordie Howe, Rosa Parks, Casey Kasem, Peter Falk, Aaron Copland, Perry Como, Glen Campbell, Eddie Albert, and Jimmy Stewart. Many others and their families have not disclosed a dementia diagnosis for fear of the stigma that Alzheimer's is a mental illness. It is not. It is an organic, degenerative disease of the brain, just as there are maladies that affect other organ systems of the human body. It must be that the brain is the organ that we most associate with being human (though I think the heart achieves that distinction as well, if primarily metaphorically).

One figure whose decline interests me is the great British mystery writer Dame Agatha Christie. While never formally diagnosed with Alzheimer's, reports of her later behavior seem to indicate it. More compelling was a textual analysis of her work by psycholinguists at the University of Toronto. They compared her later novels to her earlier ones (she wrote more than eighty books). For instance, in the later works the vocabularies of the beloved sleuths Miss Marple and Hercule

Poirot decreased by 30 percent. Overall, Christie's syntax and word choices became simpler and more repetitive. Researchers concluded that the earliest sign of the disease could be found in her writing long before it manifested much later in her observable behavior. Of course, this has spurred me to start comparing my earlier writing with my current output, looking for signs that I too have lapsed into simple sentence structure and reduced vocabulary. Let me know if you've noticed. Or if I'm overcompensating.

In 1985, President Ronald Reagan signed a proclamation designating November as National Alzheimer's Disease Month. It is possible that even as he signed the document, the early pathology of his Alzheimer's had already begun. He would die of the disease nineteen years later at age ninety-three. His wife, Nancy Reagan, shared her husband's struggle publicly and helped build national awareness of Alzheimer's as a growing problem among the country's elderly and their families.

Alzheimer's is a disease of cognition insofar as it ultimately undermines our ability to think, to reason, to form cogent thoughts. Simply put, thinking is a process that requires the brain to connect bits of stored and external information. That cognitive connective tissue is disrupted by the disease. But it is the demolition of memory that we mostly associate with Alzheimer's, which may explain why it is the health threat that Americans over the age of fifty fear most. Cancer, heart disease, and other medical conditions kill more. Yet we dread the specter of Alzheimer's above them all.

• • •

WHAT IS IT ABOUT THE LOSS OF MEMORY that so unnerves us? That makes us worry that we are losing our mind at the merest memory lapse? At its most elemental, memory is our greatest adaptive survival tool. It is how we store information. Memory allows us to perceive danger as well as recognize opportunity. It distinguishes friend from foe. It aids us mightily in predicting the future.

Memory also directs moral behavior. It is where we store the knowledge of right and wrong and how to apply those standards to our own behavior and that of others.

But it is intact memories themselves that illuminate our past, a light we shine on our lives, our library of stories. Memories tell the story of who we are, our joys and our sorrows, our triumphs and failures, our loves and our heartbreaks. They're a road map through life. Our memories are like a mirror. We peer into that mirror and see ourselves reflected in it. Do we fear that with Alzheimer's we might one day look in the mirror and see nothing? Or as Lear laments, "Who is it that can tell me who I am?"

Or is there something, something permanent? Is love a feeling? A memory? A memory of a feeling? Or is love something indelible that even Alzheimer's can't defeat?

Descartes averred that, "I think, therefore I am." But can we also say just as surely, "I love, therefore I am"? Love is not a thought, though we think about love—a lot. It is not an emotion. Emotion is how we experience love, but it is not love itself, just as the scent of a rose is not the rose.

I don't know if anyone has ever fully captured the essence of that universal source of wonder and human fulfillment. Shakespeare and King Solomon perhaps came closest. But even the sonnets and the Song of Songs fall short in that they must rely on the imperfect mechanism of language to describe something that transcends language, that words and imagery, no matter how lofty, can only approximate. Certainly, God's love is ineffable. We recognize it without truly understanding it. We are not meant to understand it.

Which is how Alzheimer's could cast a light on the permanence of love, the barrier against the complete loss of self we fear Alzheimer's occasions.

continued on p. 24

· · ·

THROUGH THE YEARS that I have been editor-in-chief, *Guideposts* has published many moving stories dealing with Alzheimer's, primarily from family members and loved ones. This is a disease that attacks every kind of family—happy ones and dysfunctional ones and all those in between.

Love is what holds families together, often imperfectly, sometimes painfully. After all, your family is one thing you can't change. Which is why the story Patty Rose told in *Guideposts* in 2009 about her troubled relationship with her father has stayed with me as an example of the primacy of love and its redemptive power, even in the face of Alzheimer's. Tolstoy said, "All happy families are alike, but every unhappy family is unhappy in its own way." Nothing could be truer than the story Patty told about her and her father.

Patty's father was a hard man, critical and controlling. As soon as she was old enough Patty moved as far away as she could and had as little to do with him as possible. Not that she didn't think of him. She did, but almost always with anger, bitterness, and resentment. She could never care about such a man, or even pity him. Love him? No, he had seen to that.

Patty had built a life of her own, marrying a man so much the opposite of her father, a man who was kind and loving to her and their daughter, who understood her pain and accepted it as a part of the woman he loved. It was as if she had created a whole new identity for herself, building the life she had hoped for growing up, and found something she could give herself to. Perhaps not healing—for there were wounds that would never completely heal—but acceptance. The family she had with her husband, Dennis, was an answer to the cruelty of her own upbringing, a sanctuary from her father and the memories that couldn't quite remain buried. After all he was her father, and she could never change that or the feelings that go with it. Some feelings just don't fade even with time and distance.

The memories were as vivid as yesterday. Patty's dad was a Marine and never let you forget it. The first song Patty learned as a toddler wasn't "Happy Birthday" or "Jesus Loves Me" but "The Marines' Hymn," and she had better sing it out or she'd have to do it again and again until she did. It seemed like he was never satisfied.

"He ran our house like a military barracks," she says. "Everything by the book and the book was whatever he said it was." He fought with Patty's mom constantly, and their sniping and bickering and screaming matches were the soundtrack of Patty's childhood, a cacophony she couldn't shut off. In bed at night she would cover her head with her pillow to drown out their angry voices. Anger seemed to be at the heart of everything. *Why can't you just love each other?* Patty thought. *Didn't you ever love each other?*

She remembers at Christmas having to hang the tree ornaments just so. They had to be perfect. Invariably her father would tear them all down and rehang them so there was exactly the same spacing between them. "Can't you do anything right?" he'd sneer.

Language is so much a part of what makes us human, liberating our thoughts and feelings for better or worse. It is how we connect…or not. And it was what Patty's father didn't say, never said, that scarred her the deepest. "If I could have heard him say just one 'I love you, Patty,' it would have made all the difference, given me something to hang on to. But he never did. I prayed and I prayed but I never once heard those words." Words every child needs to hear.

She simply couldn't understand why her father was so hard and unloving. Why? What had made him that way? He was like a man encased in armor who thought his family was the enemy. On practically the day she turned eighteen, Patty told her father she never wanted to see him again and left home for good. A few years later, so did her mom.

And that was that, until one cool winter day when a call came from the manager of a trailer park where her now-aged father lived, about 500 miles away in Southern California, on the colorless outskirts of the desert. Surprisingly, perhaps, he'd given Patty as the person to contact in case of emergency. *Why*, Patty thought as she held the phone in her hand. She didn't know.

"Mrs. Rose," the manager said, "there's something seriously wrong with your father and, well, you know, he ain't got no one. Would you mind coming down here and checking on him?"

It had been a long time since Patty had last seen her father, and she only wished it could have been longer. Part of her wanted to cut the call off, the way her father had cut her off emotionally, cut him off once and for all now that he needed her, payback for all that pain. Who could blame her?

Staring at the phone, momentarily paralyzed, she felt an awful chill ripple through her, like a cold wind from the past, drawing her back. He was her father—a terrible one, yes, but family all the same, like it or not. He was in trouble and there was no one else to help him. *But why me, Lord?* she wondered.

Some flicker of mercy deep within her, perhaps the price she was paying for the healing she found in her husband and daughter, kept her from hanging up. "I'll be there tomorrow," Patty heard herself promise.

All during that long drive, her heart burned with resentment, and by the time she reached the seedy old trailer park her father apparently called home she was ready to have it out with him. How dare he expect her to help him! Who was he to ask anything of her? Where was his hard pride now? What, was she supposed to stand there and belt out "The Marines' Hymn" for old times' sake? She wanted so badly to turn around that by the time she knocked on the door of the decrepit trailer the manager pointed to before walking quickly away, her hand shook with both fear and anger.

No answer. She knocked harder—it felt good, even the pain in her knuckles seemed like a relief—and then let herself in with the key the manager had told her she would probably need.

At first, she didn't think it was him, this figure in the gloom, as if it had all been some awful mistake. He sat slumped on the sofa, bent and frail, staring vacantly, no longer the rock-hard Marine whose image had been branded into her memory. Then came a look of confused recognition to his rheumy eyes.

"Dad?"

He stared at the floor. Everything was in disarray—papers stacked up everywhere, food rotting on the stained Formica countertop, a small table overturned. The stench was so bad she had to step outside for a breath and to gather herself, all those sleeping memories coming awake. When she went back in her father was crying.

He probably hadn't showered in weeks and God only knew how long it had been since he had eaten anything. Patty's heart sank. Now what?

He's family, Patty kept telling herself. *He's my father.* She tried to push away her empathy the way he had pushed her away, but it was no use. She couldn't just walk away. What kind of a person would that make her? A person like him?

He certainly couldn't remain in that rattrap of a trailer. She located his wallet and ID, packed up a few of his things, cleaned him up a bit, and took him home with her. It wouldn't be permanent, she told herself—just until she could get him to a VA hospital and find out what was wrong with him. Had he had a stroke? Then he would be someone else's problem and she could get back to the life she had made without him. *Maybe all he needs is some decent nutrition*, she told herself. A nagging voice said it was more than that.

It was. Patty's dad had Alzheimer's. "At this stage your father can no longer live on his own," the doctor told her. "I'm shocked someone didn't step in earlier. Thank God you got to him."

As the reality of the diagnosis sank in, Patty's mind recoiled. Thank God? Wasn't there some drug that could make him better? Some breakthrough therapy? Something?

No, the doctor said, that's not how it goes with Alzheimer's. There are some drugs that help some patients for some time but the disease is progressive and incurable. As the prognosis was laid out, Patty thought of a sandcastle being slowly devoured by the evening tide.

"It's okay, Patty, we'll manage," Dennis said when she brought her dad home from the hospital. *They could put him somewhere*, she thought—that's what we can do. But it felt so wrong when it should have felt so right. He deserved this diagnosis, his sad life. "I'll help you," Dennis said. "We can't just abandon him."

He abandoned me, she thought, remembering the love her father had so parsimoniously withheld, how she had prayed as a girl to hear him say that one word just once.

It wasn't the practical business of caregiving that held her back—the cooking and the cleaning, having to watch him so he didn't wander off or hurt himself or do something awful. She could handle that. It was the emotional toll that caregiving extracted. How can you take care of someone when you refuse to care *about* him?

One night she was reciting to Dennis the familiar litany of accusations and grievances against her father, all of which had erupted again now that her father was back in the picture. "He ruined my childhood! Stole it from me! He was angry, bitter, hateful!"

Angry, bitter, hateful. The words suddenly reverberated through her mind like a tolling bell. Angry, bitter, hateful. Was she talking about her father or herself? And really, was there a difference? Wasn't it all just the same feelings, passed down like some toxic family inheritance?

She'd held on to these feelings so tightly, like armor she herself had donned, that this insight stunned her to her very soul. Her father was going to die slowly, disappear into himself until there would be no hope of a reckoning. How could she let him forget what he had to done to her? *It's not fair!* As if the disease itself could absolve him.

All at once she understood that she couldn't let that happen, not if she was ever going to attain true healing and wholeness. That night, when she prayed, she asked for help and forgiveness, for understanding and reconciliation, for all those gifts she would need if she was ever to find peace in her life. It wasn't about absolution, it was about acceptance. What could be crueler than a disease that steals our memories? Our stories? Paradoxically, it unlocked those very things in Patty's dad, as if the disease had thrown open a door to a past he'd locked away, traumas the memories of which he had hardened himself against with his formidable armor. As his capacity for short-term recall eroded, it was as if Alzheimer's had pulled back the curtain and the ghosts of his deeper memories arose.

He would ramble disjointedly about his own troubled childhood. Patty had never thought of her father as a child—only a stern, unfeeling adult. Now she tried to imagine her father as a vulnerable child who was becoming that vulnerable again in the grip of a dementia that tore at his defenses. She learned that his father had committed suicide, a primal loss that he could never explain or completely recover from, a loss that would animate his life and define him as he fought off the dread that it might have been because of him that his father died the way he did. She watched him cry remembering his father. Again Patty thought: vulnerable, pitiable, innocent. Human.

With that awareness came something like forgiveness, or at least a release of the past, of the hurt and disappointment of a childhood she could never change, of the love she would never have. She could not forgive her father's cruelty, but she could finally accept who he was and what had happened to him and between them, a father she had no role in choosing, one she would never have chosen if she had somehow been given that chance.

No, it wasn't forgiveness of her father that mattered as much as her own reconciliation with herself, a step forward that would unshackle her at last from the pain of her own childhood. It was a tragedy that her father's childhood had ruined his life. It was just as much a tragedy if it was allowed to ruin hers. She could not allow herself to pity him for the life he had led or the disease that was killing him. Pity would only distance her from him, provide a soft armor. Somehow Patty would have to open herself to him before the oblivion of Alzheimer's consumed him.

Leaning over slowly as her father rambled on one day, Patty reached her arms around him and pulled him close to her. She held on like that for a long time, for the first time, crying softly into his shoulder, and thinking, *You are my father and there is not much time.*

One evening Patty brought her father his dinner tray. He had been eating very little lately and speaking even less, and most of what he said made little sense, his mind lost in the haze of Alzheimer's, a haze that is like some briny fog of the sea that thickens at night. Soon they would have to move him to a care facility that could do more for him than what she and Dennis could, not that much more could be done, really. There is a point where nothing can be done, except to wait on God.

Outside the sun was setting, its dying rays slanting through the blinds, casting shadows like slots on the floor.

> As Patty put down the tray, her father's frail hand reached out and took hers. She could sense him trying to summon the strength to grip her tightly and pull her closer; she could feel the weakness of his pulse. The words came slowly but clearly, as if from the depths of his soul. "Thank you for taking care of me. I love you, Patty."

I SAID EARLIER THAT IT IS THE HEART that makes us human as much as the brain. Maybe more so. For centuries philosophers and poets believed that the heart—that diligent pump—literally ruled our thoughts and our lives, the very repository of our humanity. Isn't it amazing, then, how Alzheimer's allowed Patty and her father to break free from the pain they shared and find the love that was always in their hearts, occluded and elusive, but the one thing the disease couldn't steal?

In hearing from readers on this subject, time and again they have said that love endures even the ravages of dementia. I remember my mother smiling at me as she was dying, her caregivers slipping ice chips through her parched lips, the only palliative care we would consent to at that point. Was she just reflexing at the sensation of the cold or something else? Her eyes moved toward mine. She hadn't spoken or eaten or walked or anything that constituted living in a long time, but that smile was nothing if not love, love when everything else, even the process of thought itself, had been extinguished. Love is not the process or product of thinking. It is something far more enduring, something inextinguishable. When God breathed life into us He breathed love. For that is what life is at its essence.

It may seem odd, then, that my mother did not say "love" easily. The word was not spoken regularly in our household. She came from a tough-minded, competitive Irish-American family—three boys and three girls and two strong-willed parents who carried the family through the Great Depression. If you said it first she would answer in kind, almost automatically, and I knew she meant it. Still, it came out more like a word than a feeling. "Of course I love you, dummy. Now don't be late for the school bus." Love was an assumption.

• • •

THERE WAS ONE TIME WHEN SHE SAID IT differently. I was about ten, the summer after my brother Bobby died, something I will talk more about later. Dad was out of town on business, as he often was. The day had been cloudy and threatening but the sun finally fought through late and I badgered my mother into taking me to Cass Lake for a swim. Because the weather had been so unpromising, the beach was deserted and the sun was already slipping away, a short day's work. Even the lifeguard had gone home.

There was a tall metal slide I liked to go down headfirst that deposited you right into the lake. Had the lifeguard been on duty he would have prohibited my headfirst technique. But since I was on my own I went for it with as much velocity as I could generate, arms outstretched.

I did something with my hands so that when I hit the water I plunged headfirst to the bottom, jamming my head into the hard sand. I was stunned but not unconscious and it took me a minute to find the surface, my mother standing at the water's edge with her hands clasped to her face in horror. My shoulders were hunched up around my ears and I had the wind completely knocked out of me. I tried to say "Mom" but couldn't get the word out.

Mom pulled me onto shore and held me in her arms while I got my breath back. "I love you so much," she kept saying, looking into my eyes. "I love you. Oh, your beautiful eyes. Are you okay? You're going to be okay. I love you. I love you so much."

The intensity of her reaction was unnerving and soon I caught my breath. My neck was sore, but that was about it. But I was shaken. I dried off and we went to Howard Johnson's for burgers and shakes. Mom kept checking if I was all right and ruffling my hair (I knew she was actually checking for a bump).

The next day we went to see Dr. Wilson, who pronounced me healthy but dumb. "You could have broken your neck. You're lucky it's just sore."

A couple years later I'm sure my mom was telling me again she loved me in the back of an ambulance that was hitting 90 miles an hour after I was hit by a car while riding my bike, but I was unconscious and wouldn't wake up for some time. As you can probably deduce by now, I put my mother through a lot, and this was just the beginning. But when all else failed, that word *love* took over, that word that means everything.

As the first symptoms of my mother's dementia emerged I always made it a point to end our phone conversations with "I love you." Not rote, not an afterthought. I wanted her to really hear it. And she would answer in kind, as always. I don't think I knew then how important that word was becoming to her. Something was changing in the way she said it. Yes, she was saying goodbye at the end of a phone call. But there was something more to that goodbye, a beginning as much as an end. As if denial could suppress only so much.

The Apostle John wrote, "Whoever does not love does not know God, for God is love." It is that love I found in my own journey and in the stories of others that assures me that even as the mind fades the heart lives and God is present. It is a theme I will come back to many times in the chapters ahead.

• • •

As I said earlier, love is what holds families together, even in the midst of illness, pain, and difficulty. Here are some takeaways I learned from Patty's story:

- **Never give up on love.** It is more powerful than anything. Patty and her father discovered that.

- **The word *love* has a power all its own.** Until nearly the very end my mother finished every conversation with me by saying, "I love you." Even our final one.

- **You can never say "I love you" enough.** Even when you don't want to say it. Dementia can cause people to behave erratically, even cruelly. I'll tell you more about some of my mother's most difficult moments, moments when it seemed that she hated us, but it was really what the disease was doing to her that she hated. Love them anyway and say it.

CHAPTER TWO

TRYING TO HOLD THE WORLD TOGETHER

My first steady job was in fact at that very Howard Johnson's where Mom took me after I nearly broke my neck at Cass Lake. It was situated at 15 Mile Road and Telegraph Road, its orange roof and turquoise steeple unmistakable. Sounds pretty mid-century Americana, right? The suburban '60s, to be exact.

I'd done many a neighborhood job before that—lawn cutter, pet sitter, pool cleaner, housepainter, house sitter, paperboy, door-to-door miracle cleaner salesman. When I turned fifteen, I decided to interview with Mr. Bohanic, the harried proprietor of this particular HoJo's (he hated that nickname) which was in walking distance from my house on Pebbleshire Road in Birmingham, Michigan. I got hired for the summer, no doubt in part because my mother was such a good customer, her and the ladies from church.

My duties were split between the front of the house, where I bussed tables in my jaunty paper soda jerk hat with all the appropriate orange and turquoise branding, and the back of the house, scrubbing pots and loading the dishwasher. I did not think about it much at the time, but I was aware of the racial divisions in the workplace. The back of the house crew was all Black and the front of the house all white. In fact, all female, except me. I was the exception in both areas.

Order in the front of the house was kept by an older, largish waitress named Carol whom you crossed at your peril since she made up the schedules. The rest of the waitstaff was made up of girls just maddeningly out of my age range. I wonder sometimes how my life might have been altered if I had accepted their invitation to join them on a road trip to an Upstate New York music festival called Woodstock late that summer. They were pooling a portion of their tips to finance their exploit.

"My brother is letting me have his van," perky Peggy said. I liked Peggy a lot.

I had a good degree of freedom as a kid, even after what happened to my brother Bobby, but not *that* much. "Absolutely not," my father said. "You'll worry your mother to death." All I had to do was look at my mom and know I wasn't going anywhere near someplace called Woodstock. Mom was a liberal but not that liberal, as I knew from testing her every chance I got. I was one of those surprise late-in-life babies. I'm told that after my birth my mother's hair turned completely white, which my siblings still claim I had much to do with.

• • •

ON WEEKDAYS, HoJo's WAS A BREAKFAST SPOT FOR folks who had attended 8 a.m. Mass at St. Owen's around the corner—the church where not long before I had been an altar boy. They came in groups, but we were always ready for them, mostly older folks, retired and such. It was beyond the reach of my adolescent imagination to think of ever reaching that stage of life, especially since, as I've mentioned, I did not really know my grandparents. I wish I had. Grandparents play such a formative role in their grandchildren's lives, not the least of which is helping them to appreciate the continuum of life and what it means to grow old.

One regular post-church group included an older couple. The husband routinely ordered for his wife and since perky Peggy was their favorite waitress and I was always eager to help Peggy, I often served the couple's breakfast.

The wife's name was April. She was always perfectly put together and made up and seemingly a typical older adult until I overheard her conversations with her husband. They were almost circular in nature, spiraling around the same thing. It reminded me of the old Abbott and Costello "Who's on First?" routine except for the quiet, infinite patience of the husband, who always reminded April what she ordered.

"April, sweetheart, the English muffin you wanted is at one o'clock on your plate."

"I didn't order an English muffin. I don't like English muffins. What are they?"

"Watch your coffee. It's at five o'clock."

"I thought I wanted tea."

"No, tea is after dinner, dear. Here, have a little oatmeal."

"Oatmeal?"

"You need something in your stomach to take your pills."

At first, I thought it *was* a kind of routine, though it didn't take much to understand April was visually impaired and her husband was orienting her using the face of a clock as reference. I went out of my way to help with their order though I'm not quite sure what prompted it besides my interest in Peggy at first. I soon found myself making sure April and her husband always had everything they needed.

One day, while clearing their dishes, I observed April closely. Not a hair out of place, not a smudge of lipstick, her nails perfect, none of which, I realized, she was capable of doing herself. Somebody did that for her. Someone cared enough to know she would care if she could. So the husband cared. A lot. The more I saw them, the more I realized they weren't to be written off as some old married couple having the same thing every day for breakfast (and probably lunch and dinner). No, there was this all-consuming intensity with which the husband looked after his wife. I think I began to understand then how profoundly one person can love another.

At fifteen I'd never really thought about older people being in love. That seemed the province of the young, all about urgency and longing, not patience and devotion. I could only imagine how much time and care it took him every morning to get his wife ready to go out to church and breakfast the way she wanted to be seen. As for himself, he always wore a pressed shirt and tie and a jacket. It wasn't just keeping up appearances. My adolescent brain somehow realized that he was trying to hold their world together.

After Peggy and her cohorts made off for Woodstock in her brother's van, Carol made sure I continued to attend to the elderly couple. Carol had known me since I was a little boy and loved my mother. Everyone in that restaurant knew my mother and her affiliation with St. Owen's, and that I had grown up with a Down syndrome brother who we'd lost just a few years earlier under terrible circumstances. I had the feeling Carol thought I needed to wait on these two. "Take good care of them, Eddie. Things aren't easy for them. You know how that is."

How had April gotten into this condition? This was a lot different than Down syndrome, and she wasn't crazy. She seemed to be trying to put some puzzle back together again. I didn't quite understand if her husband was there to help reassemble that puzzle or just help her with the fact that she never would. At the time I had never heard of Alzheimer's. Few people had. But I would.

Decades later Mom's symptoms began to emerge. She was still managing at home but having trouble remembering to make herself regular meals, especially since Dad wasn't around to prompt that activity. Joe and Toni and Mary Lou signed her up for Meals-on-Wheels. My mom, of course, was having none of it. Some people are resistant to caregiving. She certainly was at first.

"She just puts all the food they deliver in the freezer," Mary Lou told me over the phone. "She claims she's keeping it for people who really need it. We can't get her to eat any of it. She wants to give it away to the poor." I couldn't help but laugh and love her more than ever.

I left HoJo's after that summer. The acquisition of a driver's license opened whole new horizons. I never knew what became of Peggy and her merry band of Woodstockers (though I was jealous). Today I know the inevitable course April's life took. I sometimes wonder what became of her husband, though. His devotion was so manifest, but at some point, it wasn't enough. What did he do then?

• • •

WE THINK OF ALZHEIMER'S AND RELATED DEMENTIAS AS conditions that afflict individuals. True enough. But the demands these diseases place on family members and loved ones is enormous, on a scale arguably unlike any other illness. According to the Alzheimer's Association, more than six million Americans currently suffer from the disease, a number that will double in the coming decades, with a dollar impact on the economy of $355 billion by 2050 in the absence of a cure.

Perhaps the real toll it takes is on the constellation of people in the life of that patient. Currently 12 million Americans provide unpaid care to sufferers of Alzheimer's and related dementias. The math isn't hard. For each patient, two people provide voluntary care, almost always at home. This constellation of care includes spouses, children, other relatives, friends, neighbors, church members. Really, anyone whose love for the patient compels them to help ease their suffering.

Maybe because of my experience as a busboy at HoJo's, I've come to believe the hardest caregiving falls to the spouse. To see the person who has shared their life with you slowly succumb to a disease that erases their identity is to see a part of your own life disappear. You try to hang on to the memories your loved one is losing. Sometimes you hang on even when your loved one is gone.

The average life expectancy of an Alzheimer's patient after diagnosis is about eight years, though other medical conditions associated with old age impact this data. In some cases, people can live much longer, and with better evaluation tools people are being classified with dementia earlier. Remember, the underlying pathology of Alzheimer's may begin years before easily diagnosable symptoms emerge.

Who is the first to notice symptoms? Anecdotally, it's the spouse. After all, you likely rise in the morning together and fall into bed at about the same time every night. In between those hours there are countless interactions where something amiss can be seen.

How disturbing, then, when you first notice. Maybe it's a missed appointment, a confusion about the date or day of the week, a hundred different things that can be normal lapses when they occur occasionally but are worrisome when they increase and worsen. What everyone I've ever talked to has said is that confusion is the first indication that something is wrong. Our memories are so integral to how we organize our thinking that as neuronal changes occur, they manifest themselves in the execution of basic daily life tasks, or remembering what you did with those car keys, as I have blogged about.

> "Edward, don't worry about misplacing your car keys. Worry
> when you can't figure out what they're for! Don't sweat the small
> stuff." —Melanie, Portland, Maine, blog reader

Actually, that glib rejoinder is not entirely true. Dementia can start in some people with those small memory deficits, like the ones I fear in my own daily life. Don't panic! Most memory slips are nothing more than products of an aging brain, just the way your heart skips a beat every once in a while.

Still, the toll Alzheimer's takes on the spouse, from those first tentative suspicions to the heartbreaking end stage, can be nearly as impactful as the disease itself. I'm not sure my father could have dealt with it. The caregiving is all-consuming, so much that some spouses immerse their identity so deeply in it that life loses meaning once the object of their care has passed on. They become lost, despairing, and without hope.

continued on p. 43

• • •

THE AFTERMATH OF caregiving and the seeming loss of love is one of the hidden costs of dementia care. Sonsyrea Tate shared with *Guideposts* the story of her grandfather, Clifford Thomas, who struggled to go on after caring for the woman who had been the love of his life since high school.

Sonsyrea had accompanied her grandfather to the cemetery that oppressive August day in Maryland, the darkening sky seemingly ready to burst with rain. Not even the breeze occasioned by the golf cart they were riding in along the winding roads of the cemetery helped cool them. They were there to finalize funeral arrangements for Charity Thomas, Clifford's wife of seventy-six years and Sonsyrea's grandmother. They rode in silence.

I'm worried about him, Sonsyrea thought. As the driver eased the cart over a speed bump, she stole a glance at her grieving grandfather. Was he crying? No, there was a vacant expression on his face, almost as if his life had ended too, and with it any reason to go on. Charity had struggled with Alzheimer's for five long years, her husband at her side through it all. Sonsyrea hoped that with her grandmother's passing Clifford might find a sense of relief, even peace, that his wife's suffering had ended. It seemed now as if his was just beginning.

He finally spoke when they reached the gravesite. "It's a good thing you're seeing where everything is because you'll be back here for me soon."

Clifford Thomas was not a person given to self-pity. He'd come of age in the Great Depression, a young Black man in the segregated South. He'd served in the Army in World War II, his segregated unit fighting its way up through Italy and taking many casualties. Returning home after the war, he rose in the Marriott organization to become one of its first African-American chefs, holding that position for more than forty years. He built his life on self-discipline, stability, a rock-solid faith, and complete devotion to his wife, his family, and God.

His no-nonsense demeanor made Sonsyrea think he might have never actually left the military. Clifford could be irritable and demanding. He could be tough on his children, especially Sonsyrea's mother, and various grandchildren he called "rambunctious." Showing up five minutes late for a family dinner meant you were actually ten minutes late and would earn you a look you would not soon forget. He demanded that the younger generations respect their elders and keep the faith.

Her grandfather's gruffness never bothered Sonsyrea growing up. Even as a little girl she could see the tenderness and respect he unfailingly showed Charity, whom he called "Baby." The rest of it was just for show, the persona of a man who had lived a life of hardships and challenges and had undeniably prevailed.

They reached the gravesite where years before Clifford had bought side-by-side plots for himself and Charity. Now the ground around one was freshly tilled and the damp smell of earth rose from it, ready for the casket, which would be lowered in after the funeral. Sonsyrea jumped out of the cart and rushed to help steady her grandfather as he took a step toward the grave. There he stood staring bleakly at the ground. Sonsyrea tried to look beyond the neat rows of gravestones that stretched over a hilltop and into the distance. Out of the corner of her eye she saw a single tear drop from her grandfather's eye. *I'll have to be strong for both of us now*, she thought.

"Granddad, I know you feel like you were living to take care of your Baby, but the rest of the family…we need you too. I need you."

Clifford said nothing but his granddaughter thought she felt him lean a bit more into her arm as she led him back to the golf cart.

When her grandmother was first diagnosed, her grandfather repeatedly corrected his wife, especially as she became more disoriented, as if he could turn back the tide of the disease by his will and determination. "C'mon, Baby, you know what day it is. It's not Sunday. What day is it?"

As she grew worse his denial grew more desperate. "You don't need to be doing that," he'd say as Charity washed the dishes for a second or third time. "Leave those dishes alone!"

Desperation turned into frustration until Sonsyrea herself stepped in. She visited regularly in the evenings and on weekends. "Granddad, she's not hurting anything," she finally sat him down and told him. "Just let her be if it makes her feel better."

She saw the toll caregiving was taking on him, this man who thrived on order and discipline. Now after decades of a stable and fulfilling marriage he was losing control by the day, losing control to a disease, losing the connection to the woman he'd loved since high school. Maybe that's why it was so important to him to keep his beloved in their home to the very end. He couldn't bear to send her to a memory care unit. Family members tried to explain how he could share the burden with others trained in the care of Alzheimer's sufferers. He would have none of it, thank you, and everyone knew there was a point where they couldn't change his mind and trying only got them "That Look."

Sonsyrea had lived with her grandparents while she went to college. They were enjoying retirement by then, living an active lifestyle, bowling, golf, tennis, fishing, gardening, and singing in their church choir, where they had always been prominent members of the congregation. In the evenings the three of them would play dominoes. Sonsyrea's grandmother would bring out her old dented pot and pop a batch of buttery popcorn while Granddad would mix a pitcher of Country Time lemonade.

Then it was game on. Big time. Sonsyrea and her Granddad really went at it. They played to win and laughed loudly and boasted about running up the score. That's right, they trash-talked dominoes. It was so intense that Charity would eventually say, "Y'all take the fun out of the game," and head up to bed with a laugh and a wave of her hand. I think she knew how much alike Sonsyrea and her grandfather were.

Sonsyrea knew a spirited game of dominoes was not going to pull her grandfather out of his despair now. It wasn't only grief and exhaustion he faced but also his own health issues. His left ankle swelled. The skin on the bottom of his feet peeled off. Every day he took thirteen medications in addition to prescription eye drops. Yet with all those health problems of his own, he still put Baby's care above all else for all those years. He had home healthcare aides himself, but when he grew irritable or impatient and wouldn't take his meds, Sonsyrea was who they called.

"Look, Granddad, you gotta stay strong to help Grandma. You don't want to end up in the ER or worse. What would she do then? You fought so hard to keep her at home."

He'd relent to his granddaughter's entreaties, but grudgingly, because that was the kind of man he was, even if it was just a point of pride. Now Grandma wasn't there as a source of motivation, as his purpose. Now there was nothing.

After the funeral, she drove her grandfather home from the cemetery in silence. *What if I lose him too, Lord?* she worried. *I'm not ready for that.* After the funeral she told her mom how concerned she was.

"We can't let him give up on life like this," her mother agreed. "We have to convince him we need him to stay here with us until God calls him home." She shook her head and closed her eyes. "Lord, we have to be his purpose now," she whispered.

Life has a way of complicating matters. Sonsyrea had just gone through a divorce and started a new job. Her life was up in the air. Her mom stepped in to take on the caregiving her grandfather needed, though he was uncooperative. He constantly asked what reason he had to go on. Why keep taking all these pills?

Sonsyrea called him every day and visited as often as she could, trying desperately to find ways to break through to him.

"Whatcha doing?" she'd ask when he picked up the phone.

"What do you think I'm doing?" he'd say, sometimes with a sigh, sometimes with the sharpness of
a snapping turtle. "Ain't nothin' *to* do. I sit here and
watch TV and the TV watches me." Watching court-
room reality shows—as if searching for some pocket of
fairness and justice in the world now that his world had
collapsed—and old cowboy movies where the hero
gets the girl and they live happily ever after and no
one gets Alzheimer's or has to take thirteen pills a day
plus eye drops.

"Grandma wouldn't want to see you like this," she
said one day.

No answer.

"Why don't you check out the senior center?"

"You kidding? I don't want to hang around a bunch
of old people. You hang out with a bunch of old people
and you end up just like them—old. No siree!"

Sonsyrea couldn't suppress a smile. Her grandfather
was knocking on the door of 100. Was there a hint of the
old feistiness in his voice? That flinty contrariness? The
grandfather she'd known all her life? Was he messing
with her?

More than a year had passed since that oppressively
hot day in the cemetery and Sonsyrea's life had settled
down, so she could visit more regularly now. She noticed a subtle shift in her grandfather. The sadness was
still there, yes, but it was receding. One night, Sonsyrea
stopped by after work and said, "You ready for me to
whip you at dominoes?"

"It's a deal. But you ain't whippin' nobody, least of all me. See ya next Friday."

On Friday her grandfather met her at the door and led her to the dining room where a home-cooked meal of fried chicken, cabbage, and corn bread was waiting. The man was ninety-nine! The old chef still knew his way around the kitchen. She remembered how he always made sure his Baby had her favorite foods and proper nutrition during her decline. It was something nobody else could do for her.

Afterwards Sonsyrea cleared the dishes and her grandfather set up the dominoes. Then they got down to business. "I'll keep score," Sonsyrea said, "'cause you gonna need all your energy to try and beat me."

"That's why I fed you, girl, so you wouldn't have any excuses about being hungry or something."

They played furiously until it was near midnight. "This game is for the championship," Sonsyrea announced, glancing at the clock. They were neck and neck at this point, only one domino left for each of them. In the end, Sonsyrea had the winning play.

"I let you win," her grandfather said. "If I don't let you win occasionally maybe you won't come back."

There was a gleam in his eye, almost a tear, but brighter, alive.

"I still miss her, you know, every day, from the minute I get up."

"So do I, Grandpa."

"I miss taking care of her."

"You took great care of your Baby."

"And now God is taking care of her," he said. "I just decided to give it all up to God. He'll take good care of me too. I just got to trust He will."

Sonsyrea thought back to that gray day in the cemetery and how her grandfather had seemed to give up, had wanted to go into the ground with his beloved wife. She was afraid there was nothing she could do to bring him back from the precipice of his grief, grief that can be a kind of grave too. That tenacious stubborn streak made him so difficult to deal with sometimes. Yet it also gave him the spiritual fortitude to fight his way through the loss of his wife to a pernicious and baffling disease, and nearly the loss of himself.

The whole extended family turned out for Clifford Thomas's 100th birthday party. He was resplendent in the white three-piece suit the deacons in his church had given him as a gift. They all spent the evening roasting and toasting him and naturally Clifford gave as good as he got. Six months later he even took to the dance floor at his church's Christmas party, the crowd going wild.

In 2020, at the age of 101, Clifford died, a victim of the Covid-19 pandemic. At long last he would be reunited with the woman he cared for and loved so fully.

THE STORY OF CLIFFORD AND HIS GRANDDAUGHTER SONSYREA recalled for me that man we left back in HoJo's. Did he move on with his life after April died, as she surely did within a few years? There was so little support for family caregivers back then, and even less understanding of the struggles they faced. Then there were people like my mother, who resisted caregiving, who saw it as surrender. It was a delicate dance to get her to accept the help she needed. She could be as stubborn and contrary as Clifford ever was.

Moving on from caregiving can be complicated, an ambivalent passage. The caregiver can feel guilt—especially survivor's guilt—depression, remorse, social disconnection, loneliness, and a lack of purpose or direction in their lives. The death of one you have loved and cared for leaves a gaping hole in your life.

• • •

Our friends at Home Instead, whom Guideposts has partnered with on several content efforts, offer a number of strategies for coping with what I am calling post-caregiving burnout. I've included some of my own suggestions.

- **Reach out to family and friends.** They will share in your loss even though you may have grown distant from them as caregiving consumed more and more of your life. Renew the relationships with those you love and who love you. Trust that they will understand and support you.

- **Stick with your support group.** If you've enjoyed the community of a caregivers' support group, consider staying on. Your experience, strength, and hope will be an inspiration and source of encouragement for others. Also consider joining a bereavement group. Many churches and synagogues have them. The people you meet there will likely have been care-givers themselves and are facing the same challenges. You can't and don't have to start this new chapter of your life alone. The temptation to isolate can be strong and will keep you from moving forward with your life. Fight it.

- **Take on a new challenge.** This could be a hobby you've always wanted to try—learning a language, cooking lessons, dance lessons, singing, or simply volunteering in your community. Make yourself available. Once you're back on your feet, think about travel. Make a list of all the places you've always wanted to go—near and far—and start going. Travel can change your life. Discovering a new place to live isn't such a bad thing either. Find your new horizons.

- **Exercise.** You've probably neglected this aspect of your life during caregiving. Hike, bike, run, walk, swim. Join a gym. Get moving. You don't need me to tell you the benefits of physical activity. I will point out that in addition to building a strong body, it's also the best thing you can do for your own brain. Every study ever done on the subject has found that regular exercise increases brain health.

  I may have overdone it, actually. At about the time my mom was diagnosed, I discovered a new indoor exercise craze called spinning, an intense aerobic biking program. There weren't many classes at the time, but I found every one of them. As the craze grew so did my addiction. I'd ride two, three times a day and eventually got my instructor's certification and, years later, a new left hip after more than the equivalent of 100,000 miles of cycling. The irony is not lost on me that I didn't actually travel anywhere at all. At the time I didn't understand how much my obsession with riding was really me trying to outrun my feelings, smothering them with feel-good endorphins that are released when you compulsively drive your heart rate to anaerobic levels. I tried to explain indoor cycling to my mom once. The only thing she could think of to say was, "Well, just don't get run over by another car again."

- **Put yourself out there.** Keep the people you love close and never forget to tell them the place they hold in your life. And not just the people you love. Make sure to do the things you love—concerts, movies, the theater, museums, a walk on the beach. Seek out others who enjoy the same things. Make new friends. Bring all the love you can into your life. That is how you heal and attain spiritual well-being. Or as Dave Grohl sings, "It's times like these you learn to love again."

Most of all, trust your faith. In twelve-step groups they say God stands for Good Orderly Direction. Trust and you will be led.

CHAPTER THREE

CAREGIVING FROM A DISTANCE

When I was seventeen I left my home in Birmingham, Michigan, for the University of Michigan, Ann Arbor. I'd applied to a lot of colleges and had gotten into a few of them, some that my father favored over Michigan, but I'd always had my heart set on being a Wolverine. Ann Arbor was only an hour away by car, but in terms of vibe and overall culture it was a different world altogether from the staid northern suburbs of Detroit.

I never moved back to Birmingham, not that I didn't know I could and would have been welcomed. It simply seemed that once I left that house on Pebbleshire Road, there was no going back. My life lay ahead of me, not behind. I always moved forward. I craved the freedom of the future.

Besides, my parents were getting older and closer to retirement, and they had earned their right to peace and quiet after raising four kids. Why re-inflict myself on them other than at holidays? My mother, of course, never missed an opportunity to invite me to visit, but whenever I went home, I worried about her battle with psoriasis. She had it all her adult life and it tormented her. She used to scratch holes in her clothes trying to quell the intense itching. Of course, she refused medication, especially steroids and creams, which were the standard treatment at the time. I'd watch her standing behind the breakfast counter in our kitchen, her arms going up and down, scratching. It seemed like Mom never went more than a few minutes without scratching. No wonder her clothes had holes.

The only cure she sought was warm sunlight. She loved the beach and cruising, and it really did help, if only temporarily. Michigan's long gray winters didn't, however. Then something miraculous occurred: Once I left the nest, her psoriasis practically disappeared. My sister thought it might be due to the change of life, but I think it had as much to do with having raised her children and finally seen them off on their own. She was angst-free. Why would I go back and trigger more scratching? I used to kid her about it and her only answer was, "Well, I guess the Lord finally answered my prayers."

• • •

IN THE YEARS THAT FOLLOWED I LIVED ALL over: New Mexico, Connecticut, Massachusetts, New Jersey, New York. Yet I always found a sense of security in knowing that my parents were only a plane flight away in an emergency. Even during the months I spent wandering remote regions of the Southern Hemisphere I knew I could get back if I had to. Imagine the years before modern travel when leaving home could mean months, even years, to get back, if at all.

Surprisingly, one of the earliest signs of my mother's troubles was that she turned me from a Detroit Tigers fan into a New York Yankees fan. Please don't boo. Hear me out.

I am—or was—a born Philadelphia Phillies fan due to the fact that my mother was a born Phillies fan. She was devoted to all the Philadelphia sports teams but none more than her beloved Phillies. She watched every game and was rarely off her feet, pacing and talking to the players through the TV screen (and occasionally the umpires), clapping her hands and often clasping them in prayer. No shame at all in praying for your boys— Don Demeter, Richie Allen, and the sainted Robin Roberts.

Yet truth to tell, devotion can be transitory. We moved to Detroit in the early '60s. The internet was still just a gleam in Al Gore's eye. No cable yet, and certainly no internet. There were only three national networks, and they didn't show local games. How could Mom keep up with her Phillies? She needed a team to root for. So, she fell in love with the Detroit Tigers and all the other Motor City teams...but especially the Tigs. And so, of course, did I. The team would go on later that decade to win the World Series—Mickey Lolich, Willie Horton, Al Kaline—a trophy denied the luckless Phillies since the Truman administration.

When I went off to Ann Arbor for college, most of my weekly phone conversations with Mom had at least one mention of the Tigers. It was de rigueur. I received an artist-in-residence grant in Taos, New Mexico. Once or twice every week at my general delivery mailing address arrived a package containing the Detroit sports pages that always had coverage of the Tigers, even during the winter interlude known as hot stove season. Those pages of newsprint stuffed inside often haphazardly taped manila envelopes with Mom's scrawled return address in the corner—she had dreadful handwriting—were my lifeline, not just to a team I loved but as a way to anchor me when I felt lost and uncertain about the future and had started down the path of alcoholism and addiction.

The Detroit sports pages kept coming when I went East for graduate school and followed me down from New Haven, Connecticut, to New York. And it was there that those sections from the *Detroit News* and the *Detroit Free Press* started to break my heart. Sometimes they weren't the sports pages at all but the financial sections of the papers. Or the Living section. Or something completely irrelevant and bizarre. She'd call and say, "Ed, did you change your address? I just had a package returned to me." Of course, Mom had addressed it all wrong and it was the saddest thing to have to explain that to her, sadder still because she would stubbornly argue about it. Not because she had a point to debate. She was arguing against the fear that her mind was slipping.

• • •

EVENTUALLY THE ENVELOPES STOPPED ALTOGETHER as Mom's condition worsened, though I'd still look for them, hoping against hope, praying a prayer I knew would not be answered the way I wanted it to be answered. I'd think about how she'd go to the Franklin Post Office, a little hamlet that boasted a sign that said, "The Town That Time Forgot." (Generations of scamps had ritually altered "time" to "brains.") She'd drive the oversized Monte Carlo my dad left when he died, peering over the steering wheel, her prematurely white hair making her look like a Q-tip driving the car.

Concurrently—and possibly because of losing their greatest fan—the Tigers fell apart. They played poorly, indifferent to losing. At one point it looked like the team wouldn't make payroll and would have to be bailed out by the other major league teams. It was an embarrassment. Ownership stopped caring. And so did I. I could no longer love the Tigers, not without Mom, not with what they had turned into, and not without my sports pages in the messily taped manila envelopes that had followed me around the country for so many years.

And there was this young team in the Bronx with exciting home-grown players—Derek Jeter (a fellow Michigander, by the way, and nearly a Wolverine), Bernie Williams, Jorge Posada, Andy Pettitte (upon whom my wife formed a crush). In a strange way, this bold and talented young team gave me hope in a very dark time, something to root for. My mother always hated the Yanks, but this version of the team was not the result of the profligate free agency signings of the past, as if ownership was playing with Monopoly money but usually buying damaged goods.

So, I became—and remain—a Yankees fan. They are my true hometown team now. I have inherited my mom's need to root. In 1996, four years before my mother died of Alzheimer's, the young Yankees improbably won the World Series. Three days after Opening Day that year, I had my last drink, by the grace of God. Somehow this transference of team loyalty felt like a kind of transition in my own life, which is why I am telling you about it.

Not long before Mom could no longer live on her own, I flew back to Detroit and took her to a Tigers game. We sat in the hulking green ballpark on Trumbull Avenue on a cool sunny day, getting there early so we could hear the smart crack of the bats during hitting practice. I don't know who the Tigers played or if they won. We left early because Mom was cold, and I knew she was tired and having trouble following the game. So was I. I was thinking of the finality of life and the passion of a true fan and how it lives in the heart, nursed by unending hope. As I helped her up the stairs to the concourse she stopped and turned for one last look at the sun and the shadows and the impossibly green grass. I hoped it was a memory she would never lose.

• • •

WHERE DOES ALZHEIMER'S BEGIN?

In the brain, of course, perhaps years before acute symptoms appear, because Alzheimer's is an organic disease of the mind. There are competing theories on what actually causes the intellectual functions of the brain to decline in this manner, especially memory, but it is known that rogue proteins play a significant role in the deterioration of brain cells whether as a cause or a result of the disease.

It can also begin in families. If you have a parent or sibling with the disease, recent research indicates you are more likely to develop Alzheimer's. Genes likely play some role but exactly how is still not fully understood, though mutations on four genes involved in the production of beta-amyloid proteins that contribute to the plaques found in the brain cells of Alzheimer's patients postmortem is an area of intense study. However, people with no first-degree relatives with Alzheimer's can still succumb to the disease. Diet and environmental factors are also suspected in playing a role. Obesity, poor sleep patterns, and anxiety may also contribute. Typical Alzheimer's may involve a combination of factors.

However, there is a rare form of familial Alzheimer's that causes early-onset dementia and is known definitively to be genetically inherited. The research into the genetics of this form of the disease may yield insights into classical Alzheimer's. Only about 1 percent of all Alzheimer's cases is this rare heritable form.

You can argue that the disease really begins when we notice the earliest symptoms in ourselves or others. This morning I couldn't remember if I took my daily vitamin. Is that a bug or a feature? By which I mean, is it a symptom or just the normal misfire of an aging brain or any age brain? Not a single organ in my body is as vital as it was thirty years ago. Entropy trumps everything.

I had a drama professor who liked to invoke the word Greek philosophers used to signify when a character in a Greek tragedy ultimately recognizes his true nature or the true nature of another person or dilemma: *anagnorisis*. In other words, the conversion of ignorance to knowledge.

• • •

THE FIRST TIME I FELT THE COLD REALIZATION that there was something more amiss with my mother's mind than just a fluky memory was on a visit home one summer in the early '90s, when Mom was still mailing me an occasional sports section. Julee and I both had a break in our schedules, and we wanted to see my mom's new house.

Earlier that year, my brother Joe and his wife, Toni, had arranged to buy the home next door to theirs, a sweet little house that reminded me of an English cottage, and move my mom there from the house she'd lived in for thirty years on Pebbleshire Road, which had more space—and stairs—than she needed. Plus, the proximity of the new house made it far easier for them and my two nieces, Clare and Rachel, to keep an eye on Mom. All in all, it was a wonderful if temporary solution.

Julee and I flew out with our adorable young cocker spaniel, Sally Browne, so Mom could meet her new grand-dog. Mom had taken care of a lot of dogs in her life, including my beloved boyhood poodle, Pete, and we figured she'd be a good match with Sally.

"Maybe we should think about getting her a dog," I mentioned to Julee.

That, I soon realized, would be a terrible mistake, especially for the dog. Looking back on it today I wonder how I could have even considered it. Yes, I'd been receiving troubling messages from my family, but my mind had filtered out much of that information or rationalized it.

We were blessed with several days of perfect early summer weather. And indeed, Sally and Mom were fast friends. They shared many qualities—they were both tough, proud, independent, and stubborn.

The first night around the dinner table I complimented Mom on her new house. Mary Lou, Toni, and even Clare and Rachel had done a wonderful job decorating it, bringing over most of Mom's furniture, and getting her a few new pieces, which she sorely needed. I mean, she still had the hi-fi and set of statement mirrors she won as a TV quiz show champion, to say nothing of the threadbare couch she and Dad couldn't be bothered to spend the money to replace. Both products of the Great Depression, they were anything but pretentious or profligate.

"This place is perfect for you," I said. "Hardly any stairs and very cozy."

"It's quite nice but I'm not sure what was wrong with the other place," she said.

"This is more manageable…"

"I thought I managed the other place…"

"Pebbleshire."

"…just fine."

"Toni and Mary Lou went to a lot of trouble."

"They didn't have to."

More than anything my mother never wanted to be a burden or a bother to anyone. Nor did she wish to appear ungrateful. This move, though, was a sore point despite what I tried telling myself. Mary Lou had said that when they initially broached the idea with Mom, she'd been amenable to it. As time went on, she procrastinated and made excuses. Finally, Mary Lou and Toni more or less took matters into their own hands and got it done.

"Well, you'll get used to it," I said.

"And look at that yard," Julee added. "It's huge."

Mom smiled. "It's a nice yard and I'm sure I'll get used to the house."

"You'll be closer to the girls, and they can drop by whenever they want," I said.

Mom nodded. She wasn't really buying my argument.

"I'm just not sure why all of this was necessary," she said, getting up to clear the dishes.

For an instant I thought that maybe she did understand, on some level. That she recognized this as a possible prelude to what would ultimately be a loss of independence, where decisions about her own life would be taken out of her hands. A woman who declined membership in Mensa because she thought it was pretentious.

We helped Mom with the dishes, then the four of us—Sally too—went out to sit on the patio and gaze out on Mom's new backyard. I was happy to see that her bird feeder and St. Francis statue had come along from the old place. I grew up with those two favorites of Mom's. Sally made a beeline for St. Francis, sniffing at the base. Our previous cocker, Rudy, used to lift his leg on poor St. Francis, much to our horror. Mom would just laugh and say that of all the saints, Francis wouldn't mind.

We talked as the soft sunlight gave way to dusk and the fireflies emerged, flickering points of light. Julee loved fireflies almost as much as she loved talking to Mom, so we sat for a long time until the air grew chilly, and we decided it was time for dessert.

• • •

THE NEXT DAY I TOOK JULEE ON A tour of my childhood, as it were, showing her Wing Lake, where I played hockey, the self-consciously modern St. Owen's circa the 1970s, where I was an altar boy, and Wylie E. Groves, where I went to high school. That night we all went out to dinner—Mom, Julee, Mary Lou, Toni, Joe, the girls, and me. I felt a little nervous leaving Sally behind in a strange house. In a few days I would feel the same way about my mother.

Dinner was fine and so was Sally, though happy to see us return, especially Mom.

"They're really hitting it off," I told Julee.

The next day we did a little shopping at a mall I hung out at as a teen. When we returned late that afternoon, I went to feed Sally her dinner. We'd brought an ample supply of her food with us. I was nevertheless alarmed to see how the supply had dwindled. We'd left Mom instructions on feeding Sally while we were out the last couple days. It dawned on me what was happening.

I glared at Sally, waiting for her dinner. "What are you trying to pull?" I hissed.

Her stubby remnant of a tail vibrated. *Who, me?* Sally was sweet but she was shameless when it came to getting food out of humans. It was her life's mission. Evidently, she'd convinced Mom she was starving and having forgotten if she had fed her—and being inherently a soft touch—Mom kept doling out the kibble. No wonder they were getting along so well!

"Mom, how often are you feeding Sally?" I asked, trying to sound casually curious.

She evaded the question by opining that Sally was still a growing dog and was I hungry for a snack. "I made some cookies." I knew she hadn't made any cookies. She'd bought a bag at the bakery at Farmer Jack's grocery and transferred them to her own container. Did she remember or did she think she actually baked them?

I explained the situation to Julee. "I'm worried Mom can't remember if she fed Sally, so she just keeps dumping kibble in her bowl and sharing an apple with her. Sally has caught on. She's conniving. She's taking advantage! We have to put a stop to it."

"Calm down," Julee said. "I'll put her stash in my luggage and we'll leave out just what she's due in little baggies while we're out."

The next day, I told Mom about the new system, trying to sound nonchalant. There was a chilly pause.

"I know how to feed a dog," she snapped, and I thought of all the times she fed Pete when I should have been doing it but was too busy with hockey or band or something else.

How strange that first moment is when you overrule a parent, when the very dynamic of a lifelong relationship reverses, like the magnetic poles of the Earth flipping. I watched Mom in the kitchen, her back to me, fussing around. I knew she was angry and humiliated. Was she scared? Was she thinking of her sisters? Or was she in denial? Talk about ironclad. Mom's denial was positively bulletproof. My mom was from proud Irish-American stock and there is little the Irish fear more than losing their minds.

• • •

IT WAS AT THAT MOMENT, FOR THE FIRST time, that I was afraid for her. And for myself. We were so much alike. Would there come a day when I, too, could not be trusted to feed a dog? I pushed the panic out of my mind. Besides, it was selfish to worry about my own fate at a time like this. Mom needed our attention, our prayers, and our love.

That night, the night before we were to return to New York, Julee and I went over to Joe's house after dinner. I told them about the overfeeding incident. Toni spoke up.

"Right after we finished moving her in, I helped her plant a garden on the side of the house—plants, bushes, bulbs."

"And her roses," Julee said.

"It took most of the day, but we got it in pretty good shape. It was a good start, and I knew how much your mother loved her garden back at Pebbleshire."

I took a sip of my Diet Coke and looked around at my brother's living room. It was one of the most accommodating rooms I've ever been in, all the wall space devoted to books. We kids were all readers, thanks to our mother, who always had a book by her chair. In a way these rows of books were as much hers as Joe's, considering her influence.

"I went over the next day to check on her and couldn't believe what I saw. The garden was gone. Torn up. I looked around and saw that everything was stuffed behind the garage. So, I asked your mom what had happened. She said she had no idea. She didn't know anything about a garden."

Dear God, I thought, and if there was a true moment of Alzheimer's anagnorisis, it was then.

We spent most of the evening discussing Mom. Mary Lou said that Mom adamantly refused to have a housekeeper come in a couple times a week to straighten up and help her out. They'd tried one young lady and Mom had driven her away.

"She has good days," Mary Lou said. "Good weeks even, but then there are these incidents. And after what has happened with Cass and Marion…."

She didn't have to finish the sentence. Julee and I walked back to Mom's using the lighted path through the trees that Toni and the girls had made. Mom was asleep in her chair when we got in, a book open on her lap. I wondered how long she might have been trying to get through that book. She woke up when she heard us and said good night before heading to her room. Julee went off to call her mom and I sat out on the patio with Sally Browne, whom I had forgiven for her criminal behavior. After all, she was a dog, and sweet as could be. Even after we had taken control of the food Sally rarely left Mom's side. It wasn't just about the food. Dogs often have a sense, a mysterious ability to discern our situations. Sally knew Mom needed her close, and she obliged. It was her duty.

I sat for a long time, staring into the darkness. There was no denying any longer what was happening to Mom and somehow I would have to deal with it.

The next day Julee and I left early for our plane back to New York. We gave Mom big hugs then she bent down to say goodbye to Sally. "I'll miss you," she said, and there were tears in her eyes.

· · ·

IT WAS FOLLOWING THAT TRIP THAT THE BURDEN of distance began to weigh on me. Hearing about Mom's problems from New York was hard. It engendered a sense of powerlessness. That sense of helplessness paled in comparison, though, to the spasms of guilt I experienced every time something came up about Mom. Why wasn't I there for her? She'd always been there for me. How selfish was it of me to move so far away from someone to whom family was everything! Who else did she have besides her children? I told myself no one wanted me to pursue my dreams more than Mom, but did that matter now when her world was slowly falling in on her? Couldn't I return the love and the care she had given me? Wasn't that what it meant to be a good son? How could I leave the burden of caregiving to Mary Lou, Joe, and Toni?

Then came the cruise to Alaska. She'd signed up with a group from church. We all thought it would be a great break for Mom. She and my dad had loved sailing on cruise ships. I can still remember seeing them off at the Philadelphia docks, streamers flying, horns blasting, waving to them and my father's cousin Mac McConomy and his wife, freckle-faced Trudy, who always had champagne in their hands. After my father died, Mom took a trip to Europe with a group—my father never had any interest in going to Europe—and then to Ireland where she visited with cousins. She'd come home with some wonderful experiences and new friends.

A cruise to Alaska seemed like just the thing to keep her mind active. But Joe and Toni got a call shortly after the ship put out to sea. Mom was confused, disoriented. She demanded to be let off the ship and go home, as if home was just a car ride away. She was up at all hours of the night wandering and asking questions, talking to herself.

If I knew as much then as I know now, this would have made sense. Even in the early stages of dementia, a sudden change in location can be disorienting and panic-inducing. Couple that with the jet lag from the flight to Seattle, where the cruise originated, and you have the formula for a break with reality. Which is what Mom had. What if in her confusion she had jumped overboard thinking she could swim to shore—she was a good swimmer—then was lost to the cold waters of the Gulf of Alaska? It was heartbreaking.

I have a feeling the ship's doctor may have treated her with tranquilizers, and people in her group were able to keep her calm and oriented, but it was not a good experience and when she got home the effects seemed to linger. So did my guilt and my fear of what would come next and how would we handle it.

And especially how I would handle my feelings, from such a distance. Yes, I could fly home every chance I could but that wasn't the same as being there. Plus, there was Julee's mom, Wilma, back in Creston, Iowa. She'd had a serious stroke and Julee, too, was struggling with being a long-distance caregiver, talking to her mom on the phone every day, even though Wilma was aphasic, and going back to Iowa as often as possible. And then there was Sally and our young Lab, Marty, our newest addition. We couldn't leave them alone. They needed care. Everyone needed care! So, one of us would always have to be in New York.

It was a lot of pressure and stress, and looking back on it now I see that it was even worse than I realized or could admit. When you are in the middle of that kind of stress it is often difficult to see the trouble you're in and how you need to take care of yourself first. Julee calls it the oxygen mask principle. On a plane that may be going down, you are told to put your oxygen mask on first before trying to help others. If there is one crucial thing about caregiving from a distance it is that self-care is just as essential for you as it is for a caregiver who is on scene. You can let yourself be a self-caregiver from a distance, as it were. Learn to be good to yourself, which isn't necessarily as easy as it sounds, as I found out.

Yet many families figure it out, as mine eventually did.

• • •

ONE OF THE BEST FRIENDS *GUIDEPOSTS* MAGAZINE HAS had through the years is singer Amy Grant. In fact, her first story was the cover the month I came in for my first job interview and I was duly awed (and eventually hired!).

Amy had contributed a story to the editorial series the magazine was doing on the subject of loneliness, something we knew from our Prayer

Fellowship letters that many people struggled with. How could such a successful young singer experience this problem, though? Amy wrote that everyone suffers feelings of loneliness at some time or another, but we are never truly alone because as the Psalmist tells us God is an ever-present help. I was impressed with the maturity of this rising star's faith.

It was her story in the February 2013 issue that had the most lasting impact on me, however.

Readers tell us that they appreciate a story from a celebrity if it's about how faith helped them through a problem the reader can identify with. Readers aren't particularly interested in the vicissitudes of celebrityhood. They want a real story from a real person, heartfelt and sincere.

As an editor, I know that's what we got from Amy. Her 2013 story pulled no punches as she bared her soul about both her parents suffering from dementia: her mother was stricken with Lewy body dementia, an aggressive brain disease similar to Alzheimer's and sometimes mistaken for it in its early stages. Her father, a noted Nashville oncologist, had Alzheimer's.

continued on p. 68

• • •

AMY TELLS THE story of how she and her sisters recognized and then dealt with their parents' dual decline. She told her story so movingly and with such a depth of faith that I don't presume to be able to tell it any better, so I'm including the story from 2013 here.

My dad loved to sing and loved any meal that brought our family together. He loved boats and the beach and being outdoors. He loved God, and his prayers were filled with gratitude. He taught me how to spell my name in Morse code, to play pool and ping-pong, to bait a fish hook, but the important things he taught me were by his example. He was compassionate, caring, and respectful. I never heard him say a negative word about another person. What a lesson that was.

Dad is eighty-one now. His once-brilliant mind has been ravaged by dementia. He doesn't know my name. He rarely says two sentences in a row that make any sense. And yet without words he is still teaching me one of the most important lessons of all: how to trust God in the smallest moments, how to see that God is still present and working through all of us, even now, even on those days when I don't understand a thing my father is saying except the word "beautiful."

Dad was a respected radiation oncologist. He trained and taught at MD Anderson in Houston, Texas, and has spent most of his life in Nashville practicing at Vanderbilt, Nashville Memorial, and St. Thomas hospitals. His main work was at Park View/Centennial, which opened the Sarah Cannon Cancer Center, named for one of his patients.

When I first started my singing career, people recognized my name because of his accomplishments. They would come up to me and say, "Your father is such a wonderful doctor. He treated my mother a couple of years ago and it made such a difference. He has a wonderful bedside manner. It gave us so much confidence and hope. We'll never forget him."

Today he doesn't remember what happened an hour ago, let alone five minutes ago. He'll launch into a nonsensical conversation with disjointed phrases and I'll hold his hand, listening. He had a beautiful voice—still has—but he's lost all the words to the hymns he taught me, the ones we sang together. Sometimes I'll sing one to him and he'll pick up the tune, but if I stop, he's lost again, as if the notes just fall off the page.

"Why?" I've asked time and again, along with my three sisters. Why did this happen to this vibrant, intelligent, faith-filled man? Why did something like this happen to our mother too? There was no history of dementia in our family. Our grandparents didn't suffer from it. We had no roadmap. Mom and Dad were both in their seventies when the first telltale signs appeared—a little forgetfulness, a little repetition. But wasn't that normal with age? I forget things all the time. It can be a nagging fear if you don't wrestle it to the ground.

With Dad the confusion grew worse, then the erosion of cognition. I was visiting my parents late one evening on a break during a concert tour. My mom was wrapped up in a robe, a blanket around her feet. There was sweetness in our time together. I stood up. "Mom, I've got to go and get on the bus. They're waiting for me."

"Are you going somewhere?" she asked.

"Yes, I have a concert in Detroit tomorrow night. A reunion tour with my old friend Michael W. Smith."

"Oh, you sing?" she said with a curious smile. "What kind of songs?" I swallowed the lump in my throat, overcome by the memories of all the songs I had played just for her. "Would you sing something for me now?" she asked wistfully.

I started in on "Revive Us Again," one of her favorite hymns. Halfway through I stopped, asking if she remembered it.

"No," she said, "but I love it. Keep going." I did until it was time to get on the bus. "Can I go on the bus with you? Can I come too?" she asked.

"Not this time, Mom, but I'll be back." I kissed her good-bye and held it together until she was out of my sight.

Mom had a type of dementia known as Lewy body dementia which involved confusion and altered realities. The good news was that it was not a constant condition, which allowed us to connect with her on good days. But Dad's dementia became completely debilitating. His vocabulary disappeared. Even familiar objects he couldn't name—a telephone, a seat belt, a fork.

My sisters, Kathy, Mimi, Carol, and I have become a team, meeting with doctors and hiring caregivers (thank you, Dad, for all of your careful financial planning). Communication has been vital. My advice to every family going through this is to talk honestly with each other. The first elephant in the room was quietly retiring my dad's medical license and then not letting him drive. My sister Mimi and her husband, Jerry, moved in with Mom and Dad for a year, but they both work full-time so we still needed caregivers. We also had to explain things to Dad.

The time came when we knew it was in our parents' best interest for them to sign papers giving us power of attorney and control of their affairs. On a day when they were having lunch with Walt, their trusted minister, my sisters and I joined them at the end of the meal with the necessary papers.

My father turned to Walt. "Is this the right thing?" he asked, holding the pen. My mother, sitting beside him with her papers asked, "Am I doing the right thing?"

Walt's got a voice so comforting it's like thick caramel. "Can you see this loving family around you?" he said. "Can you see how they care? You poured love and respect into your daughters for a moment like this. You can trust them."

This reversal of roles, caring for the ones who had been so capable, is not easy. We would adjust to one change, one new wrinkle in this long downward slide, and then there'd be something new, one more loss of function, and we'd regroup. All my life I've asked God to lead me to where He needed me. Again and again He's answered that prayer. But this time there were no easy answers.

One night I opened up to a trusted friend, telling her of my frustrations, my confusion, my guilt, my sense of loss, my anger. She listened patiently, offering suggestions, lessons she had learned in the process of losing her own parents.

"Amy, this is going to be the greatest walk of faith you've ever had. You can't see the whole picture now, but each day you're going to have to trust God more than you ever have before. Day by day you will find the inspiration you need and you'll see how God is present in each moment. Give yourself the freedom to laugh and cry." And then came the words that changed everything: "I know this is hard, but this will be the last great lesson you'll learn from your parents."

Mom's health was clearly fading. Out of the blue came the idea to bring her to our house to live with us. Mom moved into my daughter Millie's room for the last three weeks of her life. I don't think we locked our front door that whole time. People kept coming and going, nurses, hospice workers, my sisters, their husbands, the grandchildren, friends. Anytime day or night, we could go sit with her, sing songs to her, hold her hand.

A few days before she died, another inspiration hit me. *We should have a girls' night in,* I thought. *Now.* I called my sisters and said, "Come over tonight. Bring ten phrases with you, things that will trigger a memory. Don't write down the whole story. The phrase should be enough to remind you of it." Even though I'm the youngest, I can be bossy!

For three and half hours we sat around Mom's bed and told stories. She never opened her eyes, but her breathing slowed as if she was hearing every word. "Mom, this is how we remember you," we said. "This is how you showed us your love. These are the stories we tell each other and we'll tell the grandkids and great-grandkids. This was the difference you made in our life." Kathy, Mimi, Carol, and I had that precious time with Mom and with each other. The next morning when the hospice nurse stopped by to check on Mom, she said, "Your mom is in transition." In less than 24 hours she was gone.

Recently I found an old video I had taken of Mom and Dad. I asked my mother three things she loved about Dad. She said, "His smile, his laugh, his voice." When I asked my dad what three things he loved about Mom, he broke down and said, "I never want to live one day without her." It's been eighteen months since Mom passed away.

These days my father lives in a one-bedroom apartment with round-the-clock care. It's working and we're very grateful to the people who are helping us, but I have to remind myself, it's only for now. Each day brings new challenges, each day is different. Not long ago I took Dad for a walk on the farm. We've got an old log cabin in the back and I took him inside, made a fire, and we sat there like two kids on a campout. "Beautiful," he said, one of his few words these days, at least one of the few I can understand. I guess if you are going to hang on to a short list of words, beautiful is a good one.

When we were through, we went outside, stood there, arm in arm, totally present, letting a late winter sun warm us. "Beautiful," my father said. I couldn't agree more.

As heartfelt and even heartbreaking as Amy's story is, there is valuable practical information throughout it in the way she and her sisters faced their situation as a team of caregivers. Here are three takeaways from the piece on how a family can work together even at a distance.

- **Communicate.** Amy and her sisters formed a team, knowing that together they would be stronger for their parents. They divvied up duties and coordinated with outside caregivers, doctors, her parents' pastor, and each other regularly and clearly. This kind of honest communication requires courage, the courage to not be afraid to face facts and to accept that you are now responsible for your parents' well-being. That role reversal is one of the most difficult aspects of caregiving for a loved one who has cared for you all your life.

- **Be present.** People suffering from dementia, especially in the middle and late stages, tend to increasingly live in the moment. Be there for them. If they get something wrong or turned around, don't correct. In most cases you can just go with it. Remember Amy's girls' night in? That was the perfect example of Amy and her sisters meeting their mom where she was in her journey. So was her walk with her dad on the farm and the peaceful time they spent at the cabin. Experts say that showing old family videos and photos is a wonderful way to interact and connect.

- **Let God lead.** As Amy's friend said, this was the greatest faith journey Amy would ever embark on and the last great lesson her parents would teach her. As difficult as it may be to recognize at times, caregiving can be an opportunity to improve your spiritual well-being. Amy asked God to lead her through each difficult day and in so doing deepened her faith. The same can be true for you.

CHAPTER FOUR

FACING MY FUTURE

Given my family history of Alzheimer's, my chances of developing it are significantly higher than average based on recent research. How much higher is what I hope to find out, along with an explanation for these nagging lapses in memory. What did I do the other day? I went to put a jar of oregano away and put it in the dishwasher until I realized what I was doing. I put stuff in the wrong place so often that Julee is always asking, "Edward, what did you do with the..." I'm lucky if I remember.

Friends chide me to chill. Forgetting stuff as you age is just a normal part of life, they say. Frankly, I would rather have a neurologist tell me that, no offense to my well-meaning friends. So, I made the appointment.

I took Amtrak down along the Hudson River from Upstate New York—not far from where Julee, Gracie, and I had retreated to the Berkshires during Covid—for my appointment at NYU Langone Health in Manhattan. They had replaced my left hip a few years earlier so I figured I could trust them with my brain. I loved the ride along the river, and I made it a point to grab a seat by the window. Today was bright but cold and the water shimmered in the sunlight.

• • •

A RIVER RUNS THROUGH IT IS A GOOD movie (based on a novella by Norman Maclean) with a great title that I relate to. Rivers have run through my life. I grew up in Philadelphia on the Delaware River with its fabled bridges that I was always thrilled and a little jittery to cross—the Walt Whitman Bridge, the Ben Franklin Bridge. It was a big treat when we had to cross one. I remember the arc of fireworks reflected in the water on the Fourth. My father kept a boat on the Delaware.

Later we moved to Detroit. I took the Boblo Boat downriver to Boblo Island, passing under the Ambassador Bridge, which connects Michigan with Canada (my brother worked his way through law school as a customs agent there). Boblo, which was technically in Canada, had an ancient amusement park that dated to the 1890s and was always a bit funky and down at the heels. It smelled of cotton candy and roasted peanuts and…well, some people's stomachs couldn't survive the rickety old roller coaster. The boat ride itself, watching the great ore boats ply the river, and the lights of houses crouched on the dark green shores of Grosse Ile, made for a good date night in high school.

A few years later, while I was still a teen, I would be crewing on one of those ore boats, the hardest, dirtiest, most dangerous job of my life. It's one of the many things I can't believe my mother ever agreed to let me do. My parents drove me to the slip where I boarded a tug. The ship I was crewing on, the *William R. Roche* (named after a former chairman of U.S. Steel), was headed downriver and moving fast with the current—the Detroit River is not actually a river but a strait, hence the oxymoron of its name (Detroit is French for strait, the French having originally settled Detroit until the British kicked them out). The tug raced to catch up with the *Roche*. They lowered a ladder from the *Roche* as the two vessels bumped and slammed in the spray, plus a rope for my seabag, and up I went, bouncing off the hull and knowing one slip and I would be dead. Making my way up the steel side of that huge ship, I'd never experienced such a merging of fear and elation. I wonder now how that alchemy might have foreshadowed other experiences in my life.

• • •

For many years now the Hudson has been my spirit river. I first got sober living in an SRO—a single room occupancy—on the far west side of Manhattan. SROs are not known for their luxury. If I pushed the dingy curtain back from my grimy window, I could just glimpse a sliver of the river between the buildings, and a little more in the distance, the town of Weehawken, New Jersey, just across the water. I liked being on what I saw as the right side of the river, given my ill-fated life in Hoboken, which I'll get to a little later. It had felt like progress.

Today the river was leading me back to Manhattan, almost like a living thing carrying me to the city I love and had fled only a little more than a year earlier as Covid ravaged the population and emptied the streets of this restless, insomniac metropolis. I'd watched in disbelief as the city shut down, the hospitals overflowed, the morgues filled up, bodies stacked like cords of wood, and sirens split the air. We'd been struck by a new disease that attacked a naïve population, a population that had no natural resistance to this novel virus first identified in China.

I looked up from my reading and out the train window just as we went under the Bear Mountain Bridge. Then came the imposing gray turrets of West Point looming on the west bank. I'd briefly wanted to attend West Point—a desire almost as fleeting as my intention to attend seminary—after reading a series of boy books about a cadet-cum-sleuth who solved all sorts of murky mysteries on the old campus and its environs. That dream ended when my brother, who actually did attend a military college, put me straight about Beast Barracks and said if I talked about solving mysteries, I'd spend my time marching in endless circles on the parade grounds until I dropped. I chose the University of Michigan instead.

Gazing at that edifice gliding by my window drew my thoughts to my mother and about how much worry was at the core of her experience of motherhood. One son wanted to attain an army commission from a military college at the depths of the Vietnam War. Another wanted to spend summers working on Great Lakes ore boats, which sink from time to time and are dangerous even when they don't. I guess she prayed harder than she worried. She once told me that worry was a form of prayer because you were being honest with God about your fears. Maybe so, but I worry that the stress I put on her as her son might have contributed to her developing dementia. There is some evidence that prolonged stress can make you more vulnerable to Alzheimer's and other brain diseases. PTSD is also seen as a culprit.

• • •

THERE IS NO WAY MY MOTHER WOULD HAVE done what I was about to do. You could not have dragged her to a neurologist. Getting her to a doctor of any kind was nearly impossible. By the time Mary Lou finally convinced her to see a GP for what was billed as a routine checkup, she failed the basic clockface test—where she was asked to simply draw eleven o'clock on a blank clockface. Mom basically repressed the whole episode. I'm sure she came up with some amazing excuse for failing the test. It just reinforced her conviction that no good could come from seeing doctors. But I believe failing that test must have shaken her. I doubt she believed her own rationalization. And I'm sure she prayed about it when she got home.

As I have said, the one thing my mother never failed to do was pray, even throughout the degradations of her illness. As my train dropped underground and entered the long tunnel under the West Side leading to Penn Station, I thought about something I had written for Guideposts devotional book *Daily Guideposts* years before, after my mother had entered a memory care facility called Lourdes and I phoned her one day.

"Is she there?" I asked Sherry when my call bounced from my mother's room to the front desk. Sherry was one of the supervisors.

"She's praying with some of the other ladies," Sherry said. It was a new Friday activity for the residents, along with shopping at a nearby mall and lunch at a favorite chain restaurant where, according to Mom, their only culinary failing was serving too much food. "The portions are too big!"

I could understand too small, but too big?

Later I got through to Mom in her room. "I called this morning, but you were busy."

"Well, I must have been praying," she said after a pause.

Strange, I thought, *that she would say that.* Sherry must have just reminded her about those morning prayers or something. Her own memory would not have done that. She rarely remembered speaking to me even ten minutes after I hung up. "Has my son called lately, the youngest one?" she'd quiz the staff. When I did call, Mom reacted with spontaneity, as if I was her long-lost child. Every conversation was a kind of reunion.

The next time I called, again on a Friday afternoon because that's when work slowed down, she said the same thing, unprompted. "I was busy praying all morning."

No recollection of the mall, no mention of the popular chain that serves excessive portions. Just prayer. She remembered that. I asked Sherry about this mnemonic oddity. "Oh, yes," Sherry explained. "The one thing Estelle never forgets is her prayers. We never have to remind her."

Of course, I thought. My mother would always have prayer, and her indomitable faith, so much stronger than mine it always seemed to me.

That word *reunion*. Isn't prayer a reunion with God? A reunion my mother never forgot.

. . .

MY TRAIN JERKED THROUGH THE TUNNEL, THE LIGHTS flickering every so often when we hit an electrical dead spot. Finally, we came to a squeaky stop at least a mile short of the terminus. *Traffic*, I thought. We were waiting for a train to clear our platform.

I checked my email on my phone. There was a message from a reader referring to one of the blogs I'd been writing about my family's Alzheimer's journey. "That was a blessed moment you shared with your mom that day you described. Hold on to it! Just keep playing the trombone." Yes, it was a blog about playing the trombone, nominally. But it was about so much more, a visit I'd made to Clausen Manor, the memory care unit my mother was in at Lourdes. I pulled the blog up on my phone and reread it.

"Hi, Mom, how are you doing?" I said, dropping my bags.

My mother glanced at the aide who was straightening her bed pillows and said, hesitantly, "My youngest."

"Yes, I know," the aide said. "He came all the way from New York to see you."

"New York? What was he doing in New York?"

"He lives there. Don't you remember?" She nodded at me and moved on to the next room on the hall. "Have a nice visit."

I had the sense that Mom was searching for my name but remembered even now that I was her youngest. Years before her memory issues set in, she adopted the technique of calling out all the names of my siblings (and sometimes the dog) before landing on mine: "Joe, Mary Lou, Bobby, Pete (the dog), ED!"

Mom pointed to a chair by a window that looked out on the bird feeder we'd brought from her house—along with the companion statue of St. Francis—when we moved her here. I helped her out of bed. She loved to watch the birds, could do so for hours, especially on a pristine spring day such as this. I moved her to a floral-patterned wingback chair and sat in the matching love seat across from it. She had a lovely little suite here at Clausen Manor, a memory care unit on the Lourdes Campus, after a couple of less than successful stops at facilities I don't care to describe. Her room was full of pictures of her family, the centerpiece being her engagement portrait with my father. Mom was posed so you couldn't miss the ring on her finger. They were so young, so beautiful, so alive, so happy, so long ago. I wondered if she missed him or remembered him enough to summon those feelings. Who was he to her now more than a decade after his death?

My mind was drifting when she suddenly asked, "Do you still play the trombone?"

What a question! I almost burst out laughing. Even I didn't remember that I had played the trombone up until about tenth grade when I quit to play bass in a basement blues band. I picked up the trombone in fourth grade. I went to a big meeting with my parents one evening in the school gymnasium held by Mr. Okin, the band teacher. "You look like a trombonist to me," he proclaimed. I have no idea how he arrived at that conclusion apart from the fact that he probably needed some poor kid to play trombone and I looked capable of lugging one around.

My doctor, Dr. Wilson, later opined that it would be beneficial for my asthma, though I don't believe Mr. Okin quite realized he was conscripting an asthmatic trombone player. I liked the slide. You could make some really weird sounds with it. So, my parents rented me a trombone—rented one because no one was under the illusion I was destined to be the next Glenn Miller or Roswell Rudd. I hung with it until high school when I just couldn't bring myself to participate in marching band. What girl would date a nerdy trombonist in a silly uniform and a hat that kept falling over his eyes? I'd get further as a bass guitarist.

Yet Mom's strange question caused a memory of mine to fall open. I was nine. It was my mom's first birthday without my brother Bobby, who'd died that year. Bobby loved birthdays. Both Mary Lou and Joe were off at college and my father was away on business. It was just the two of us celebrating with one candle that wouldn't stay lit on a homely little cake from Awrey's bakery. Mom ate only half her piece. She cleared the table and sat down to a cup of tea. Her hair had turned white in the last year. I still wasn't used to it. I went upstairs to practice.

But not for long. Something about her sitting there alone with her cup of tea on her birthday really got to me. I came marching down the stairs, my trombone blaring and blatting out "Happy Birthday," slurred notes and all. It's a good thing the windows were closed, or the neighbors might have complained.

There was a pause while I finished. Then Mom nearly knocked her tea over getting up and wrapping me in her arms with a strength I never knew she had, that any woman had. We stayed that way for what seemed like a long time, me thinking what it must be like to feel what she was feeling. It scared me a bit. It still does, the sadness she must have tried to bury with my brother. Even today, if I close my eyes, I can still feel that fierce maternal embrace, the amazing strength of that long-ago hug.

Now, in her little room filled with pictures of the past, I took her hand. She squeezed back, harder than I expected. "Yes, Mom," I said because I couldn't say no, "I still play the trombone."

"Good," she said. "You were a good player."

Her eyes drifted back to the feeder and the squabbling birds until she soon slipped off to sleep. I wondered if she dreamed, or if she could still dream, since dreams are memories, perhaps not exact ones but at least facsimiles of memories, reflected in the funhouse mirrors of our somnambulant minds. Can you dream without memories? Are your memories restored in dreams? Did

Mom pray in her dreams? For a long while I sat watching her, wondering what her mind could still process. Our memories are a maze we wander. In Alzheimer's, does that maze grow smaller and more confusing and lead nowhere? But sometimes there is a little God-given miracle of memory, an image with meaning and stark emotion that breaks loose and is true in its essence. A trombone, a birthday, a hug. It happened as a shared experience for both Mom and me that day.

• • •

I LOOKED UP FROM MY PHONE. MY TRAIN had finally pulled into the platform at Penn Station with a jerk. I grabbed my stuff and headed up the escalator, taking two steps at a time, to the main concourse and out onto Eighth Avenue. I'd been in and out of the city quickly a few times during the pandemic lockdown but not for a while, and after all these months in the Berkshires, it felt reassuring to breathe city air again, even through a mask. The streets weren't exactly deserted, but they were a long way from how I remembered them pre-pandemic. I hadn't seen the city like this since 9/11. The virus had peaked for now; people's fears hadn't.

My apartment was only a few blocks away. It was good to be home, though the place smelled musty and unlived in. I opened a few windows and ordered the pad thai I'd been craving from the restaurant down the street. They were still doing deliveries.

I came in early to get a good night's sleep before my appointment, leaving Julee and Gracie behind for this foray. It was anything but. I tossed and turned. What would the doctor say? What kind of exam would he do? What kind of tests? I knew there would be tests of my memory and cognition. What if I failed? What if insurance didn't pay for all this? Did I set the alarm on my phone? I refused to let myself check. I knew I did. I didn't forget. I worried that I had lost the address even though I'd written it down and put it in my phone in two locations. Could I get a cab? Should I plan to walk? You name it, I worried about it, especially what I would do if the diagnosis was bad. Or if there wasn't a diagnosis. Was that worse? To be left in diagnostic limbo? *Well, Mr. Grinnan, we just don't know what to think about you.*

But I remembered one thing—the doctor's name, Joel Salinas, M.D. When I made the appointment, NYU Langone had randomly assigned me a neurologist in their memory and Alzheimer's evaluation center. The doctor's name struck a bell, so I looked him up and was nonplussed. He had been described in a profile I'd seen as "the neurologist who feels your pain—literally." Empathy was his superpower.

Amazingly, a few years earlier we had interviewed him for our *Mysterious Ways* magazine, and he had been good enough to do a Guideposts Facebook Live chat for us. I didn't associate him with NYU at first because he was at Harvard when we worked with him.

Dr. Salinas is a synesthetic, meaning he has a neurological condition known as synesthesia that causes him to perceive each of his senses as a mix with one or more of his other senses. Hence, he may hear colors, taste sounds, even experience people as numbers. It is a strange condition for sure. Yet he functions brilliantly and is, not surprisingly, the world's foremost expert on the subject. A feature of his synesthesia is called mirror touch. He can physically feel what people around him are physically feeling. If you pinch your left arm in his presence, he too might feel the sensation of that pinch in his left arm. Touch your cheek and he too will feel his cheek touched. Likewise, that sensitivity extends to the feelings and emotions of others as well. We had interviewed Dr. Salinas for an article we were doing on empathy. Synesthetics are the ultimate empaths, the result of a simple "wiring glitch" in their brains, as Dr. Salinas describes it. What does that tell us about the malleability of our brains?

That I would be randomly assigned to Dr. Salinas was hard to accept as mere chance. Sometimes a coincidence is just a coincidence, a random event, a product of a purely statistical outcome. Was this? No, it couldn't be, I told myself. Or at least I didn't want it to be. It had to be more. And with that I fell fast asleep.

• • •

I HEADED ACROSS TOWN FOR MY APPOINTMENT ON a blustery April morning, walking fast into a blinding sun. At this time of day and this time of the year in Manhattan, the sun is right in your eyes if you're going east, the rays glancing off the East River maximizing the glare.

By contrast, the building I entered in the East 30s had subdued lighting and it took a moment for my eyes to adjust. I showed my ID to the man at the reception desk. I proffered my vaccination card, but he waved it away and pointed to the elevator bank. "Second one."

At the appointed floor I was ushered into a small, windowless office, well-lit, with a slightly claustrophobic feel and just a few accents of NYU purple on the gray walls as an attempt at branding or cheerfulness or whatever. For a second, I wanted to bolt. What was I doing here? *This is foolish. Just get on with your life!* Then a nurse breezed in and took my vitals—my blood pressure was slightly elevated, which it rarely is—and said, "The doctor will be right with you."

And he was, amazingly. I had expected to wait in nervous silence. Since we were both vaccinated, we removed our masks but didn't shake hands. I noticed Dr. Salinas had what could almost be described as a baby face, soft and unlined. He seemed relaxed and personable and immediately put me at ease. He took a seat at a computer desk, and I reminded him of our previous association and thanked him.

"Yes, I remember. I enjoyed it. I'd just released my book."

He was referring to *Mirror Touch*, his fascinating personal account of synesthesia.

We got down to business. He asked my highest level of education. I told him. He took a medical history, including my family history of Alzheimer's and other diseases, which I related in detail, especially my mother's history, then revealed my own fears. I found myself envying his typing skills. He typed very fast as he asked questions, pausing only occasionally.

"Tell me about your memory problems."

I told him about what I called my micro-memory lapses, what neurologists sometimes classify as implicit memory. "I forget things I did seconds before—" and my concept of a computer program that runs in the background that isn't functioning as well as it once did. "Does that make any sense, Doctor?"

"Yes, I think it does. It's how you are experiencing it."

He typed some more, very fast. I could have finished this book by now if I could type like that.

"I do strange things sometimes. Like the other night when I started to use the key fob from our car to open the front door of the house. I know the fob can't do that, but I found myself doing it anyway, like I was watching myself watching myself."

He looked up for a moment.

"I went to return some oregano to the spice cabinet and opened the dishwasher instead. I almost put it in before I stopped myself. I open the refrigerator when I mean to open the side door to the outside. I can't remember if I applied the parking brake to the car even though I'd done it seconds earlier. This happens practically every time I park. I've even started to make lists. I never used to need lists. I could remember everything, even things that had happened weeks or months before. When I came to New York after graduate school I waited tables. I could take an order from a table of six purely by memory. I couldn't do that for three people now. My short-term memory isn't as sharp as it once was. I feel it's been slipping more and more lately. My mind drifts. I forget names a lot, names I should know. Sometimes I can't remember people I'm supposed to remember, or it takes me a couple seconds, sometimes longer, and sometimes I get people confused. What bothers me most is when someone notices. I come up with some excuse or other rather than just laughing it off and saying I forgot. Like I'm trying to cover it up. I'm defensive and irritated. I think my mom did this years before we admitted she had a memory problem." I paused. He typed. Then looked up. I liked his expression. It said, *Tell me more. I'm listening.*

"I want to know if there is any way to tell if I have pre-clinical symptoms of dementia," I said. I overheard a plaintive note in my voice.

"Are you an anxious person?" he asked.

"I can be but not usually. But I'm more likely to be anxious than depressed."

I detailed my history of alcoholism and alcohol-related seizure disorder. Like most doctors he seemed a bit surprised those symptoms appeared so early in my drinking history. I admitted—endorsed, as his notes would later put it—that I sometimes used drugs when I drank and probably came close to overdosing on several occasions.

"Do you have suicidal impulses?"

"No, not recently."

We talked some more, and I explained my worry that I was going down the same path as my mother and her sisters and that the damage that I might have done to my brain, including several head injuries occasioned by alcohol abuse, and a fractured skull when I was twelve, could make me more likely to develop Alzheimer's earlier. I told him how much that bothered me. That I was already damaged goods.

I mentioned all the crazy supplements I was taking for brain health and that got a fraction of a smile out of him as if to say, *It's your money, dude.* It was clear he wasn't going to judge me. Did I exercise? Yes, religiously.

"Are you having problems performing your work?"

"No. I think my writing and editing, and thinking, are as strong as ever, maybe stronger. I can remember a single edit I made months earlier if it fails to appear in the final manuscript. I know why I made it. Anything I make a conscious point to remember, I usually remember. It's like I remind myself in advance. It's the small everyday things, the automatic things, where I'm slipping. It's not like me."

"Does your wife notice?"

"Yes, but she's always called me absent-minded. I've never considered myself absent-minded. Not at all. I just sometimes think about a lot of things at once. I can be preoccupied, especially when I'm writing. Even when I'm not writing I'm writing. In my head. I'm always writing. Almost everything that happens to me a part of my brain is writing about it as if that is the way I process life."

He nodded. Throughout this exchange I kept my hands at my side. I didn't want to scratch my nose or anything like that for fear he would feel it. I started to yawn but stopped myself. What if he yawned too? What if my actions dictated his?

We moved on to some cognitive tests, and I was relieved he didn't ask me to do the clockface challenge. That would have indicated a level of concern that would have been quite alarming. The night before I'd been tempted to practice it until I realized how ridiculous I was being. A wave of sadness had come over me. I thought of my mom trying to draw those hands on the clock and failing. How did that make her feel? How did she process that failure? Why couldn't I have been with her instead of 700 miles away?

We started with some simple word repetitions. Then he changed the order, added words, reversed the lists. I felt my performance slipping. I was hesitating more, and we were going back over word group-ings. When it was over, he asked, "How did you sleep last night?"

"So-so."

"Do you usually sleep well?"

"Depends."

I had the distinct impression that my performance on the memo-rization tests had fallen off as the tests became more complex. Maybe that was to be expected but it worried me. As Dr. Salinas typed I felt my heart rate increasing. Could he feel it too?

We did a few more tests, this time involving imagery, which I felt pretty good about. I stole a glimpse at my watch hoping it didn't prompt him to do the same. More than an hour had passed.

Finally, he said that he would like to follow up with a blood test, an MRI of my brain, and a consultation with a sleep disorder clinic. He informed me my diagnosis was Subjective Cognitive Decline and I thanked him, though I immediately wondered if this was something you thanked someone for. We parted ways cordially and I promised to sched-ule a follow-up appointment as soon as the tests were completed. Dr. Salinas said he'd post the notes of my session in my online chart that day.

I wasn't two steps out the door and onto the street when I whipped out my phone and googled Subjective Cognitive Decline. Most of the informa-tion was indistinct, citing the symptoms I believed I was experiencing. The primary diagnostic characteristic of SCD was that it was principally self-reported and sometimes confirmed by cognitive testing such as I had just undergone. From what I could discern, it was a murky area of brain health, but the Alzheimer's Association had some troubling things to say about it, including that the diagnosis could possibly be interpreted as a pre-clinical indication of Alzheimer's. In some people, at least. Not very helpful.

I stopped into an NYU clinic to get my blood drawn—they took an inordinate amount—then decided on impulse that I should get my hair cut. I went down to see Jessica in the East Village, who has cut my hair for years. "You don't seem forgetful to me," she said. "I mean, you always show up for your appointments."

"Well, it's probably not that obvious to anyone but me."

"You shouldn't worry so much. When I worry my brain stops functioning. I can't process anything."

Afterwards I walked across 8th Street to Tompkins Square Park. The day had grown warm, and spring was at hand. This slice of Manhattan felt as if it was achieving something like normalcy. There was always a lot of energy in the East Village. I went to a lot of AA meetings down here in any number of old churches when I was first getting sober. Good sobriety and spirituality. The park was filled with dogs and children and skateboarders, joggers and tai chi practitioners, jugglers, food trucks, street folk, and a few cops. I found a bench, opened my phone, and signed into my health chart. At least I had remembered my username and password. The notes from my session were indeed posted.

I scrolled through them. The terminology was alien though I had the impression that I exhibited no gross abnormalities physically or mentally. A lot of notes about my motor skills, which seemed normal. I could tell where I fell short on the recall tests. I googled the term "perseverations." Hesitation or repetition of thought. I had several instances of them. Noted.

My protective factors were level of education, abstinence from alcohol, intellectually challenging work, physical activity, and social relationships. My primary risks were family history and recent history of memory lapses. Possibly a sleep disorder. I sensed the jury was out on the question of whether the effects of a previous alcohol use disorder, withdrawal syndrome, and brain injury could increase one's susceptibility to dementia.

Suddenly it occurred to me we had not discussed faith, which I believe is the most protective factor of all, not just from the disease itself but from the fear and apprehension that accompanies a diagnosis.

The more I thought about the omission, the more it troubled me. Shouldn't faith be part of the discussion, an essential part? I had to assume that the medical profession did not want to delve into such nonempirical matters. But still…

I signed out of my chart, and asked myself again, What was I doing? What did I want to know that only God really knew? The future? Isn't that always what we humans desire to know most? What happens next? The future may exist in some unknowable dimension; we will never be privy to it. All we have is now and the immediacy of faith, which can shield us from the fear with which we sometimes view the future. There is an anonymous quote I love that a friend once texted me: "Thou knowest the past but not the future. As to what is future, even a bird with a long neck cannot see it, only God." I assumed the quote came from the Bible, though I could never track it down, and I suspect my well-meaning friend might have made it up himself and attributed it to "anonymous" to get me to pay more attention to it.

The diagnosis didn't tell me anything that I didn't already know, and an MRI was the next step. What was I to do with this information? Drive myself crazy? I was beginning to feel my resolve falter. Maybe knowing just a little bit made me not want to know anything else.

I watched an acrobatic dog catch a frisbee in mid-air and for a split second I couldn't recall the word for the thing he was catching. A mother nursed her baby. A man and a woman played chess on a blanket in the grass. An older woman read a book I took to be her Bible. It felt good to sit here. To be in this moment. In the now. Maybe that was all that mattered.

Faith. So much of our lives pivot on this one fundamental, spiritual truth. Without it we are adrift. Sometimes faith is the question, sometimes it is the answer, and sometimes it is both.

continued on p. 97

• • •

MANY CAREGIVERS STRUGGLE with denial about the extent of a loved one's cognitive deficiencies. That was the case for Kristen Kemp, of Montclair, New Jersey, who recently told her story in *Guideposts*. It was a story I identified with and was moved by, as I know you will be too.

Her story starts with a phone call from her mother. Following college, Kristen had moved east from southern Indiana, where she'd grown up in Jeffersonville, to pursue her dream of being a writer. Landing in Montclair, New Jersey, less than twenty miles from Manhattan and a popular enclave for journalists and other media professionals, Kristen married, had three children, and built her career. But she always stayed close to her parents, especially her mother, with whom she spoke on the phone frequently and came home to visit as much as a busy life allowed. She and her mom had even taken a memorable girls' only trip to England, Wales, and Ireland. Mostly they stayed in touch through their daily calls.

This call was different. "I'm having trouble with my memory," she told Kristen. "I'm forgetting things. I think there's something wrong with me."

Kristen felt herself stiffen. Her mother's mom, MeMe, as Kristen called her, developed Alzheimer's late in life. Kristen's mom had cared for her until the end, the kind of devotion perhaps only a daughter can give. Kristen's mom was only sixty-nine, a retired schoolteacher, still as sharp as ever as far as Kristen was concerned, busier than ever too since she "retired."

"Mom," she said, "I think you're just doing too much. All your activities, gardening, and volunteering, especially at church. Maybe you need to slow down a little."

Yet there was real fear in her mother's voice, and it rippled through the phone to Kristen. She knew how much her mother feared ending up like MeMe, eventually in need of constant care. Not that Kristen's mom regretted a minute of the care she'd given her mother. That had been an act of love. No, she never wanted to burden her family, especially Kristen's dad and Kristen and her brother. Her mother dreaded becoming that burden.

"You don't have dementia," Kristen insisted even as she wondered whether it was herself or her mom she was trying to reassure, for today Kristen will tell you that fear and denial was her first response to her mother's concerns about her memory.

Not long after, driving to a doctor's appointment in nearby Louisville, Kentucky, her mom became disoriented and lost. She had to call Kristen's dad. When he finally figured out where she was, he drove to get her, and she followed him home.

"I'm going to see a doctor about this," her shaken mom told her on their next call.

They won't find anything, Kristen thought. *Mom's too young to have Alzheimer's. MeMe was older.*

Kristen had wonderful memories of Mom and MeMe from her childhood in Jeffersonville, a city of some 50,000 citizens situated on the Ohio River, not exactly a small town but a far cry from New York City.

She remembered them all sitting in a pew together at their Methodist church. For MeMe, church was as much a social occasion as anything. She loved her friends in the congregation. Sitting beside her mom, Kristen could feel the depth of her mother's faith and how it took flight in her soaring voice as she sang the old hymns she loved so much, the music coming from her heart as well as her lips, the notes as sweet as the candy at Schimpff's Confectionery on Spring Street. Her mom rarely missed Sunday services or her Bible study group. Faith was her anchor.

It was an anchor Kristen had mostly lost in her own life. Not that she had become an unbeliever. With raising three kids and pursuing a career, church had never played the central role in her life that it had in her mom's. "Your faith will always be something you can rely on," her mother had told her. "God will be there to catch you when you fall."

And now it felt like Kristen was free-falling through fear and worry and doubt. The 700 miles between New Jersey and Indiana felt like 7,000 miles. How could she care for her mother when she was so far away? What would keep them connected if her mother's symptoms worsened? She remembered how MeMe moved in with her mother, but she couldn't do that. She couldn't move back to Jeffersonville, not with three kids in school and her husband's job, and bringing her mother to New Jersey was out of the question. Her father was still in good health. He'd see to Mom. Kristen and her brother, living in Texas, would coordinate and get back as much as possible so not all the care would fall on him.

Kristen thought again about the centrality of her mom's church family and how they would lift her up both in prayer and in practice. Sometimes counting on God meant counting on your fellow worshippers. She was incredibly grateful for the support her mom could rely on.

But what, Kristen wondered, was she herself relying on? Where was her support system? God was more of a concept than a belief she could hold on to, more distant than near. Just as she had put distance between herself and Jeffersonville, she'd put even more distance between herself and God.

Often on Sunday morning Kristen would go for a walk. One of her routes took her past a megachurch. The parking lot was always full. She could hear worship music even from the street, loud and joyous. The parishioners appeared happy and energized as they streamed outside after services, hugging, shaking hands, laughing. Each time she passed the church she found herself pausing longer, drawn to the joy and fellowship, her heart aching more and more for that connection. Finally, she went inside for a service, edging her way into a crowded pew and taking a seat. Several people turned and smiled. The pastor began his sermon. "We all suffer physical and mental health crises. Believe in God, and He will produce miracles."

What kind of miracle could I hope for? Kristen wondered. After all there was no cure for Alzheimer's, no miracle for her mother. She knew better than to hope.

After the service, people—strangers—reached out and greeted her warmly. This was not the sort of church you just walk in and walk out of. Such caring lifted her soul and so the next week she went back. And the next. And the next.

Why? What drew her? Maybe it was the music. She found herself singing, like her mom long ago at their Methodist church. She learned the words to her favorite praise songs and the music poured out of her. Singing released something inside her, long dormant, a welling of feeling, a crescendo of relief, as if faith was manifested as notes on a page. Somehow, she had found her way back to something whose absence had left an unrecognized void in her life. Until now.

She joined a Bible study at the church and started praying regularly, for her mother, for strength and understanding. She poured out all her feelings, her frustrations, her fears, her grief. For the first time in many years, she felt that God was unmistakably present in her life, a presence made manifest by grace, leading her, comforting her, listening to her. She knew that the only way she would stay close to her mom was through faith. God was showing her that what was most important to her mom must now become most important to Kristen. That is how they would stay connected through what was to come.

She held fast to the support and friendship she found at church. One Sunday, she stood to the strains of a song she'd come to love, "The Great I Am." She raised her arms high, her body swaying to the music, letting the words wash over her and through her. It almost felt as if she had become more soul than body. "I want to be near, near, near to your heart. Loving the world, hating the dark." The faith that had always sustained her mother had taken root in her. She felt as if she were living in the heart of God.

Her mother declined slowly yet inexorably. The progression of the disease was unstoppable. Her dad finally hid the car keys from her. The loss of independence was devastating and only made her worse. Kristen thought it was time for her mother to go to a memory care facility, but her brother and her dad resisted.

Kristen visited as often as she could. On one of these visits, she felt the most important goal was to see to it that her mother got to church. She knew that even as her mother's mind slipped away, church was recognizable and comforting.

Their daily phone conversations, which had kept them close for decades, became more one-sided. Still, Kristen persisted. She told her mom about her kids' sports, the TV shows they were into, her writing assignments, what she was making for dinner, the songs she sang at church. Sometimes she would sing to her mom and try to get her to sing along.

Kristen had started practicing yoga, something she couldn't have imagined just a few years earlier. Anxiety is as much a physical phenomenon as a mental one, and yoga helped Kristen to ease the physical manifestation of worry and apprehension, to flush those feeling from her being. Her pastor spoke often of how faith could take the place of worry—letting go, living in the moment and trusting the future to God. Eventually Kristen trained to become a yoga teacher herself, exploring even more deeply what it meant to live in the now, to be with God in every moment.

One day she was at the yoga studio when her dad's number appeared on her cell phone. *Something's happened to Mom,* she thought, trying to quell her rising panic. But it was her dad who was in difficult straits. He'd taken himself to the VA hospital with chest pains. He was worried but didn't think it was that serious. Doctors disagreed. They scheduled quadruple bypass surgery for the next day.

Her dad was more worried about her mom. Who would take care of her? She needed companionship and watching. Her father had been her primary caregiver for some time now. Could Kristen come home? Kristen called her husband to book her on the next flight to Louisville, the nearest major airport to Jeffersonville, and raced home to pack.

On the flight she prayed for strength—for her father, her mother, and herself. She prayed for fear to be kept at bay. She prayed for the Lord's will. How many of us have found ourselves stuffed in an airline seat racing to some crisis, held aloft by prayer?

She stayed for two weeks and tried not to be unnerved by her mother's decline. Her brother came from

Texas as well. Her mom was confused and upset by everything that was happening. Alzheimer's patients react to even minor disruptions in their lives. Kristen reached out to multiple agencies until she finally found a home health care aide who could put in a full day after she'd gone back to New Jersey. She was a sweet lady, older than her parents, who were in their late seventies by then. Meanwhile she got her mother on a waiting list at a memory care center. She knew that long term her mom's condition would be too much for her dad to handle. She didn't want to upset her father by talking to him about it then but there was no doubt in her mind that her mom would need 24/7 care.

A room became available a few months later, an answer to persistent prayer, Kristen fully believed. She went back to Indiana to help with the move. They packed her mom's clothes, family photographs, and her favorite coloring books. It was a time of both sadness and relief. Did her mom know she was saying goodbye to her home for the last time? Was she scared? Those of us who have gone through this process know how those questions feel and how hard the answers are.

The daily calls to her mother had by now become fruitless so she called her dad instead. After sixty years of marriage, he needed support and a friendly voice, tenderness and understanding. Just someone to talk to.

Through it all she held fast to her faith, and especially to the friendships she had formed at church. Singing at Sunday services was now how she stayed connected to her mom. Faith had been the answer to the question of how she would not lose her mom to a disease that threatened to turn them into strangers. In drawing her back to His house, closer to Him, God had given her a way to grow closer to her mother, a communion deeper than words through a phone. Indeed, Kristen felt this was the miracle her pastor's sermon had promised, a different kind of healing, one only God could have seen.

That Christmas after her mom entered memory care, Kristen flew home. She was worried. Would her mother still find meaning in Christmas?

She was in her mother's room on Christmas Eve, getting her ready for a candlelight service at church. She dug through a pile of clothes on the floor looking for a sweater and a scarf. She noticed that her mom's closet had plenty of hangers, but her mom, who'd always been tidy, had seemingly forgotten how to use them.

"What's happening, dear?" her mom asked. Kristen sensed she was a little fuzzy on her name.

"It's Christmas Eve, Mom. We're going to church."

"We always go to such fun places!" Her mom smiled, vacantly it seemed to Kristen, and she wondered if her mom had any comprehension of the conversation. Would she even recognize her church?

She glanced at her watch. "Mom, we need to hurry. Let's find something for you to wear. It's chilly outside."

Her father, husband, and three kids would meet them at the church. Kristen was anxious to get her mom settled in a pew early, but everything, even the simplest tasks, took so much more time now and rushing her mom would only confuse and upset her. She said a prayer for patience. Sometimes I wonder if that's the prayer God hears from us most.

They found a pew near the back of the church in case they had to leave early. Kristen knew her mom might be disruptive in "unfamiliar" surroundings. It pained her to think her mom's church might now seem unrecognizable to her. Did Christmas itself lack meaning?

Her mom sat between her and her father. The music— all those old, beautiful carols—began. "The First Noel," "Joy to the World," "Angels We Have Heard on High." To her surprise, her mother hummed and even sang some of the words, that lovely voice of hers rising in praise, as if being here in church had turned back the clock. Then she held both Kristen's and her father's hands and dropped her head.

"What's she doing? Is she okay?" her dad asked.

"Yes, she's praying," Kristen said. She looked up to see tears in her father's eyes.

Did Christmas still hold meaning for her mother? Kristen didn't have to wonder anymore. She didn't have to wonder if God was with them every step of this journey, holding their hands as they now held each other's.

At the end of the service, the sanctuary went dark. They lit the candles they'd been given when they arrived. Kristen lit her mom's. Then the congregation sang "Silent Night." Her mom's eyes focused on the light of the candle she held before her, and she mouthed the words to "Silent Night," the candlelight reflected in her eyes. After the final verse she puckered her lips and blew out the candle.

"Thank you," she said. "That was beautiful."

B EAUTIFUL. NOT A WORD WE ASSOCIATE WITH ALZHEIMER'S and dementia. And yet in researching this book I have heard about God-given moments of beauty, where the soul burst forth even when the mind is failing.

Kristen's story reminded me so much of my own, especially the pain of guilt at being distant. But it also brought back a moment that occurred in my family at Christmas. No holiday mines the memory like Christmas. The holiday spirit rides on a tide of memories, resurrecting the past in the present. It's more than nostalgia. It's reaffirmation. Yet what happens to Christmas for those whose capacity to remember erodes?

I remember a time late in my mother's illness when she was living at Clausen Manor. That year we had decided it had become too taxing on my mom to take her from Clausen to Christmas dinner at my brother's house about ten miles distant. Physically my mother, who was a runner into her seventies, was declining due to osteoporosis and congestive heart failure, the latter a common late-stage complication of Alzheimer's. Moving her was a delicate proposition. So too was the effect it had on her mind. A change of environment, even from a familiar one to another, could cause an unpredictable reaction and agitation. No one wanted to risk that.

December 25 was very cold, the way it should be in Michigan on Christmas. Julee and I had flown in from New York a few days earlier.

We had been rewarded by a fresh blanket of snow and below freezing temperatures that kept it pristine. In New York City the snow looks like frozen dirt.

Joe, Mary Lou, Toni, Julee, and I—along with nieces Clare and Rachel and my cousin Carol—piled into various vehicles and headed out to Clausen to see Mom. The facility coordinator said she was expecting us, which I knew was just a figure of speech at this point. No doubt they were telling Mom every two minutes we were on our way. "Does Mom even realize we're coming? Does she even know it's Christmas?" I asked Julee.

"At some level I really believe she does," Julee said. Julee's mom's stroke had mostly left her without the capacity for organized speech. Yet Julee had an astonishing ability to understand almost anything her mom, whose mind was sound, was attempting to say or communicate. The staff at the nursing home out in Iowa—Julee's a Midwesterner like me—would regularly call her in New York or wherever Julee was in the world to interpret her mother's wishes. Once they called her in Japan while she was doing an interview. Julee calmly took the call, listened to her mother, then said, "She just wants you to ask the woman down the hall to turn down her TV." And she was right. (I can imagine Wilma nodding her head in exasperated concurrence.) So maybe Julee possessed some insight into my mother's consciousness I lacked. Maybe she just had more faith in a mother's maternal nucleus.

• • •

STOMPING THE SNOW OFF OUR BOOTS, WE FILED into my mother's memory care facility, which was decorated with holly and candy canes and tinsel. An artificial tree with LED lights stood in a corner and carols played softly on a sound system. A staffer wheeled Mom from her room to a common area where we all could fit. It was unnerving to see Mom in a wheelchair, a recent development. Not so many years ago she would have been out shoveling snow on a day like this. The smile on her face when she saw us pushed all that aside. "See?" Julee whispered.

Clare and Rachel had brought chocolates for my mother's secret sweet tooth she always denied having. Julee and I brought a plant that I knew Mom would water to death before the New Year if left to her own devices. Cousin Carol put a fancy *Twelve Days of Christmas* pop-up book in Mom's lap, which I bristled at. I thought it too juvenile for my mother.

Yet it was Carol's present that caught Mom's attention as she sat silently in her wheelchair. We were all chatting and thanking the staff and wishing them a merry Christmas when out of nowhere Mom began to read aloud. "On...the...first...day of...Christmas, my true love...gave to me..."

She looked up and smiled. We stared in astonishment. Mom, who would read at least one book a week through most of her life, had long lost the capacity to read.

On she went, struggling. "On the second day...of Christmas my true...love gave...to me..."

To be sure, turtledoves turned into turtle dolls, hens into hills, maids into moms, but no one dared stop her. By the tenth day Mom was clearly tiring. I started to help her with a passage when she suddenly shot me a sharp look I hadn't seen in some time and snapped, "Are you going to let me do it myself?"

I almost jumped back. Then a moment of stunned silence gave way to laughter, save for Mom, who cast us a strangely knowing look. She let the book close, apparently having forgotten she'd been reading it. Did Mom know it was Christmas? For that bright, shining moment we all did.

It would be my mother's last Christmas.

• • •

ONE ASPECT OF KRISTEN'S SITUATION I IDENTIFIED WITH strongly was that we were both long-distance caregivers. The advantage, of course, was that we were removed from the daily burden of caring for a loved one with Alzheimer's. The price you pay for that is guilt and remorse. My sister, brother, and sister-in-law were increasingly consumed by the attention my mother's illness demanded and it worried me that I was not doing my part.

Of course, it was not feasible or even necessary for me to move back to Michigan and be part of the care team. No one expected that of me, even if I sometimes expected it of myself. Being at a distance made me feel a loss of control, as if I wasn't doing as much as I could.

• • •

There are 34 million Americans caring for an aging parent and roughly 15 percent live an hour or more away. About a third of that number are caring for a parent with dementia. Many feel the way I did—inadequate. This only makes the situation worse and hampers the caregiving you are providing.

Here are some tips from my own experience as a long-distance caregiver:

- **Stay in touch.** If your loved one can still hold a conversation, if only briefly, don't be afraid to pick up the phone and call. I found out that my mother was clearer in the morning than later in the day, so I timed my calls for then. One of her caregivers at her unit told me that even when she couldn't maintain a coherent conversation my mother liked hearing my voice. "She always smiles when I hold the phone up." That helped me overcome the anxiety.

- **Send cards.** The same caregiver told me many residents love getting cards in the mail, even if they don't remember who they're from. "Even if it's just for the moment, it brings a spark to their day." Such a small thing but I felt better every time I dropped one in the mailbox.

- **Keep informed.** If you have family members like mine who are close by to your parent or loved one, be sure you keep the lines of communication open. You may not be on scene, but you need to know what is going on and how you can help.

- **Plan your visits.** Look at your calendar, then block off times when you can travel to see your loved one. Let people know these times are important and can't be changed.

- **Pray.** Prayer knows no distance.

CHAPTER FIVE

ASSESSING THE DAMAGE

This is where my story might appear to take an unwelcome turn, but I would not be writing honestly if I failed to follow its path into some of the dark corners along the way that might shed some light on my current dilemma, so I pray you bear with me. It starts with this question: Does alcoholism, or a history of alcoholism within your family, increase the chances of developing Alzheimer's? I've always said that everyone has a *Guideposts* story. So instead of including another person's story in this chapter, I will tell my own.

There's an obvious personal interest here since I have disclosed earlier that I struggled with alcoholism and drug use for years starting in my early teens, when I first put that cold rim of a purloined bottle of Old Granddad bourbon to my lips and decided I wanted to feel the way this sublime substance made me feel—imbued, somehow illuminated—all the time. And for a good twenty years I tried. I chased that fleeting scintilla of ethereal bliss. The more ardently, then desperately, I pursued it, nearly to the exclusion of everything else in my life, the more elusive it became. It grew painfully clear that that moment, that feeling, transformative as it was, as transfiguring as it seemed, could never by its very singular nature be recaptured and the pursuit of it would destroy me. I took that first drink, but all the rest took me.

I told this story and how I was ultimately led to *Guideposts* in my book, *The Promise of Hope: How True Stories of Hope and Inspiration*

Saved My Life and How They Can Change Yours. Maybe this would be a good time for you to stop and read that book.

I'm kidding, of course. Please keep reading on.

• • •

THERE IS SOME IRONY IN THE FACT THAT my first drink was Old Granddad. If Alzheimer's runs along my maternal line, alcoholism comes from my father's side. He himself was not much of a drinker, most likely because he saw what alcohol had done to his father, my grandfather, whose demise was hastened by his drinking. Like so many adult children of alcoholics, my father was beset by anxieties and fears, phobias and compulsions, as well as numerous health conditions—ulcers, hypertension, heart disease, obesity, diabetes. I only wish I understood when he was alive that alcoholism is a family disease that reverberates through the generations in different ways. I think I would have felt more compassionate than distant toward him. He died just a few months into my first serious attempt at sobriety, in January of 1984, of a massive coronary while swimming laps at a Jack LaLanne health club, trying to get healthy. He was seventy-three; he'd lived longer than doctors expected him to live after his first heart attack some twenty years earlier.

Those attempts at sobriety had grown more frequent by my late twenties. I'd been expelled from graduate school for a year until I could figure out what to do with myself. A mentor—in truth, I was unmentorable—helped me reenter the program. I spent the last half of my final year living in the Yale student health service, being let out for classes only after my morning dose of Antabuse and Librium.

Where was God in all this? It was a question I had long since stopped asking. I had never actually rejected God or religion, nor had I drifted from it. It was more as if the bottom had simply dropped out of my spirituality at some point amidst my drinking and all that went with it. I can't tell you when I stopped believing that there was a God who cared about me or about anything. If there was a supreme being, He was an indifferent one and we wanted nothing to do with each other. I had no notion of an all-knowing, all-powerful God. A cosmic dictator. If anything controlled my life it was alcohol. Ergo alcohol was God. I remember once calling up AA and politely asking if they could direct me to a meeting where nobody talked about God. They put me on hold and never came back on.

It would have broken my mother's heart to know this, so we never really talked about it. Irish-Catholic families are very adept at that style of denial. Yet I knew she worried. She wanted nothing more than for her kids to know God. There were many times I felt guilty about the blackened state of my soul—and, of course, guilt is a handy excuse to drink and drug and everything else.

If there was a miracle in my life at that time it was that I managed to earn my degree, an MFA in playwriting. After I graduated, I moved from New Haven to New York, then Hoboken, New Jersey, where things went from terrible to worse. There weren't many want ads looking to hire playwrights and the jobs I did get I had trouble holding onto, mainly because I had trouble showing up, including eventually to jobs like washing dishes at a seafood restaurant in Hoboken where Frank Sinatra once liked to eat.

I also had trouble holding on to places to live, which eventually had me bouncing from friends to flophouses to the street. Penniless, I hustled change in downtown Manhattan and around the Hoboken train station, once suffering the humiliation of asking a person for a spare dollar before I realized he recognized me from the grad school dining hall. There wasn't a hole deep enough for me to crawl into.

And maybe that was the problem. My bottom seemed bottomless. There was a strangely detached spark of objective consciousness that seemed to stand back and ask, "How bad is this going to get?" And still I kept drinking, occasionally sobering up long enough to get a job and lose it.

• • •

ALCOHOLISM IS A PHYSICAL DISEASE AS WELL AS a mental obsession, and alcohol is as physically addictive as any drug you can imagine; it affects every cell in your body. Over time the brain is essentially conditioned to interpret the cravings for a drink as a survival imperative and reacts violently when denied, as if the body is being starved of essential nourishment.

I don't know exactly when I started experiencing the DTs—delirium tremens—and withdrawal seizures. They can happen without you knowing it. One minute you're sitting on the edge of the bed and the next awareness you have you're standing at the kitchen sink trying to remember what day it is and where you are and why there are bruises on your arms and legs. It can take several hours or even days for your scrambled neurons to come back into alignment.

I remember one seizure in particular, if remember is the word since a seizure wipes out your memory of it. Rather I should say I remember the circumstances. I was staying at a friend's apartment in Hoboken, sleeping on the floor and quickly wearing out my welcome. It was a bitter January day, an icy wind slicing across the Hudson from Manhattan, whose skyline nearly blended into the dreary winter grayness like an unfinished canvas. I'd been blackout drunk for a number of foodless days and now I was sobering up involuntarily due to lack of funds and a general failure of my body to accept any more alcohol. It is dangerous to come off a binge so abruptly, but I was not about to turn myself in to an emergency room. I'd seen too many of those lately. I needed a drink, but my temporary roommate knew enough not to keep anything around. I was out of cigarettes as well and would have been quick to collect a few half-smoked butts off the street next to the stoop, but I was too afraid to go outside.

I was pacing the freezing, nearly furniture-less apartment in a state of suffocating anxiety when the phone rang. I picked up and heard the voice of my best friend from Michigan, Michael, who was establishing his legal career in Manhattan. If there was anyone I could talk to in this state it was Michael. I tried to say something coherent but couldn't.

"Never mind," he finally snapped, "there's nothing to explain except that this has got to stop."

"It will," I said, with little conviction.

"How? When you end up freezing to death in some doorway? Howard found you passed out on the street the other night. You're lucky. I might have kept going."

I thought about it. I knew he wouldn't have. But would I have wanted him to? Isn't that how Poe died? Wasn't freezing to death a pretty good way to go? They say you feel paradoxically warm at the end. Some people claw at their clothes... There might have been a burst of light. I don't know. Something like a lightning flash.

The next thing I was aware of was a harsh pounding on the door. I was sitting on the edge of a chair, the phone nowhere to be seen, holding one of my shoes. I was very confused. There were abrasions on my hands and a little blood, and some fluid stains on my shirt. The light hurt my eyes. I stared at the door. It appeared to me like one of those doors in an old cartoon, pulsing and heaving like a bellows from the battering it was taking. *I better answer it,* I thought, *lest they break it down and I'd have even more to explain.* That would surely get me thrown out and back on the streets.

I limped over and opened the door meekly. Two huge cops stood there looking peeved. They too seemed to be out of an old cartoon. Giant men with bulging chests and big badges. I wondered what I had done. It had to be something. Most of the last few days were a mystery. I was ready to plead guilty to just about anything.

"Yes?" I said, my voice distant and quavering. My hands shook so I shoved them in my pockets. I didn't want to appear any more guilty than I felt. I looked at their Hoboken Police Department-issued name plates. Dunn and Rodriguez.

"Are you all right?" It was Rodriguez, who seemed the younger. It wasn't so much a question as an accusation. "We had a report."

"Of what?"

"Someone reported a scream," Dunn said, not making much of an attempt to hide his effort to peer past me into the apartment, nosy Irishman.

"It's just me here."

"Did you scream?"

"Not that I know of."

"Someone called us from New York," Rodriguez said, jerking his head in the direction of Manhattan. "They were talking to you on the phone. Then you screamed. He said it was like a shriek."

"Allegedly," Dunn added.

"I can't imagine it was me."

At this point two young EMTs clattered up the steps with bulky medical bags, eager to get to work.

"Wanna get checked out?" Rodriguez asked.

"No," I said, trying to clear my head and piece together the events of the last twenty minutes or so. "You can go."

I swung the door shut, wondering if they'd kick it in. All I heard was them stomping down the stairs, their radio squawking. I needed to call Michael back but now I couldn't remember his number or the name of the firm where he worked, two things I knew by heart. For a moment I couldn't remember his last name. It would come to me in a few hours, but I was very weak and more anxious than ever. My mind kept going in and out of focus and it was a few hours before I calmed down and called Michael back and told him I was all right.

"Oh no, you're not, Edward. You better come to grips with that before it's too late."

These episodes increased: the hideous shriek, the alcoholic seizures, the coming to like drifting up through the murk from the bottom of a lake right before you ran out of air. Sometimes I'd end up in an ER with a Valium drip in my arm and a doctor shouting at me to recite my social security number and DOB so he could send me on my way. Once there was a spinal tap since no one seemed to believe a person as young as me could be having such end-stage symptoms. Must be a brain tumor or something just as grim. I met an equally alcoholic doctor in a bar one night—he told me the shrieks were a common prelude to an alcoholic seizure, which was a slight relief to learn—who palpated my liver right there on the barstool.

"It's hardening and a tad enlarged," he diagnosed, then tried to get me to examine his by comparison. "Mine's worse," he said. "Feel."

Obviously, Michael was right. This couldn't continue if I expected to survive much longer. Despite not having an actual home, I wasn't truly homeless. There were my parents back in Michigan and my brother and my sister. There was a course of action. Unsteadily I made it to the PATH station.

I was almost too dizzy to make it across the vast concourse of the World Trade Center north tower, past the mammoth escalator banks descending hundreds of feet into the depths of the New York City subway system and the PATH trains swooping under the river and back to New Jersey, the sheer scale of the place obscured in the movie-effect collapse years later. My objective was a seemingly endless bank of shiny pay phones embedded in a wall, reflecting the space

I was trying—and eventually succeeding—to traverse. I saw a fun
house image of myself picking up a receiver and reversing the charges
to Michigan to the only person I could turn to. "Mom," I said, "I
need to come home."

The next morning Michael—of course his last name had long
since returned to me by now, O'Neill—drove me to Newark Airport
on what was quickly becoming a miserably hot summer Saturday. I
was woozy and hung my head out the window like a cocker spaniel.
He bought me a ticket and marched me to the gate. I tried to detour
toward a concourse bar, but he redirected me, then stopped and recon-
sidered. I guess he didn't want me screaming on the plane.

I managed to get admitted to a rehab in Lapeer County, up in what
Michiganders call the thumb. It lasted the appointed twenty-eight
days, and I had my first real introduction to the twelve-step program
of Alcoholics Anonymous, not that it took. At least not then, not
entirely, but incipiently, though I didn't actually realize it yet.

I returned to New York and to drinking but not for long. I was living
in a walk-up tenement in Little Italy that an old friend, Lisa, had vacated
to move in with her fiancé, a drummer in an up-and-coming rock
band. There was still a month or so left on the lease, so basically I had
permission to squat there while she moved her stuff out. One day she
found me leaning over the bathtub in the kitchen—it was one of those
layouts with a communal toilet down the hall—trying to drink rubbing
alcohol cut with grenadine and sniffing glue off a wad of Kleenex. She
dumped the dregs of a sixteen-ounce Olde English Ale over my head,
fired the can at me with surprising velocity, then pulled me to my feet
and dragged me all the way across town through a teeming rainstorm,
smacking me over my head with her umbrella when I faltered, until we
got to Perry Street in the West Village, where she shoved me through an
unmarked door into a room of people listening to a speaker at a table up

front flanked by sayings like "Let Go and Let God" and "One Day at a Time." I didn't know it, but I finally had a home.

• • •

I HAD FOUND SOBRIETY, OR MAYBE IT HAD found me. I didn't care. Somehow, as I was hanging over that grimy bathtub in that old walk-up, I knew I had to have God in my life. It was the only answer, whether I liked it or not. God. Jesus. Higher Power. Good Orderly Direction. It didn't matter. Just something greater than myself, the only thing greater than my addiction.

I got a sponsor. Two, in fact. I moved in with another guy in the program, Bob, who is still a friend to this day—and still sober. After waiting tables for a spell at a place that drew lots of celebrities (maybe I'll tell you about them and their tipping habits someday), I got a job as a PR writer for a venerable old Danish trading company and did reasonably well for a couple years until on a research trip to Copenhagen I somehow forgot that I was an alcoholic and picked up a drink. That is the madness of alcoholism.

I don't really think I forgot I was a drunk. What I forgot was God, deliberately and willfully. The next few weeks were a nightmare of solitary suicidal drinking and drugging, with Interpol out looking for me and my poor mother working her fingers to the bone saying the rosary, something it has taken me a long time to forgive myself for, if I ever have. Knowing now what I know about Alzheimer's, she was almost certainly experiencing the first, inchoate symptoms of the disease, which only added to her anxiety.

Early on someone called Michael and said, "We don't know where Edward is or what he is doing."

"Maybe you don't know where but don't kid yourself. We know what he's doing."

That's Michael for you.

I will not go into the miraculous "white light" experience I had sitting on a windowsill of a hotel room forty-two floors up with my legs dangling over the abyss and a drink in my hand, not caring which way I fell if and when I passed out. The phone was ringing from the front desk because my American Express card had finally been exhausted and two mysterious individuals claiming to be from Interpol were knocking on the door, much more civilly than the Hoboken cops. Yet once again I was undeservedly rescued by a power greater than myself. All of this has been covered in that earlier book. Those two claiming to be from Interpol? There is no record of them ever finding me. To this day I assume they were angels with very convincing credentials.

I managed to get back to New York. I experienced my last seizure on an unconscionably hot spring day on the West Side, in front of a Greek restaurant on Broadway. Some well-meaning soul dashed out and slipped a spoon in my mouth while I convulsed, which really isn't something you're supposed to do, except in the movies. With my head and knees bleeding, I got carted off to St. Luke's Roosevelt Hospital, admitted, detoxed with the merciful help of Valium, and CAT-scanned. I checked myself out a few days later before they could administer a spinal tap. I made sure to call Mom immediately to let her know I was alive.

"As long as you're okay," she said. "That's all that matters. I love you. No matter what. And God loves you."

I spent virtually every hour of every day in AA meetings, counting my days, studying the Big Book, and trying to humble myself before God. For it was humility that was most required. Humility and surrender. As a counselor in rehab once said, "Edward, in a not uncharming way you are incredibly willful."

Then two amazing, inexplicable things happened. Walking across West 72nd Street, right near the Dakota where John Lennon was shot just six years earlier, I encountered a woman who stood out like Technicolor against black and white. She had a corpulent cocker spaniel on the end of a leash, and I managed to insult the woman almost immediately with an ill-advised comment about the dog's weight. "He looks like the Marlon Brando of cockers." It was an inauspicious start to a relationship with the dazzling woman who would become my wife.

Not long after, I got a call from an employment recruiter who wondered if I would like to interview for an editorial job at a magazine called *Guideposts*.

"Guide what?"

"*Guideposts*. I'm looking at your resume and you might be a good fit."

I wasn't sure what she thought I would fit into. Did I want to fit into anything? Could I? I'd never heard of *Guideposts*. Also, I'd never heard of this recruiter either, let alone sent her my resume, such as it was. How did she find me? Anyway, *Guideposts* sounded like a travel magazine and that interested me. Maybe I'd get some free trips out of it—not to Denmark, of course, I'm not sure they'd let me in.

I still wasn't certain this wasn't some scam or a cult. I showed up for the interview in a painfully contemporary office tower on Third Avenue and soon realized that *Guideposts* was a magazine featuring true stories of hope and inspiration written by its readers for some four million subscribers, founded by the author of *The Power of Positive Thinking*, Dr. Norman Vincent Peale, and his wife, Ruth, in 1945. I was hardly a paragon of positivity.

I don't know why they hired me. I wouldn't have hired me. I vowed to stay only for a year, maybe less, and work on my resume before they found out more about me. Yet if you substitute the word *journey* for *travel*, that's what it's been for me at *Guideposts* for thirty-six years, one year at a time.

. . .

I BURDEN YOU WITH THIS SORDID HISTORY BECAUSE all these years later I am sometimes haunted by the fear that I may have damaged my brain in some way that would make me more susceptible to the family curse. Besides the convulsions, I incurred at least several concussions, starting with my face being driven through the glass front of a cigarette machine in a bar by a couple of testy bouncers. My then-girlfriend's father was a plastic surgeon, and he pinched the laceration above my left eye tightly and painfully closed for a good hour so I wouldn't have a scar and so that I would remember the pain. At the time he guessed I might have a slight concussion.

Later in New York I tumbled down some stairs and fell face-first through the plate glass door of an apartment building where I was staying on Park Avenue while I ghostwrote for a famous novelist who was at least as bad off as I was. The doorman was not amused, and my head ached and throbbed for days. You can still detect tiny scars on my nose. There were several more unexplained facial bruises and scalp stitches, to say nothing of the fact that I fractured my skull being hit by a car when I was twelve and was later beaned in Little League by a huge kid, Greg Konopka, who had a wicked fastball and little control. I lay sprawled in the batter's box for several minutes until I regained consciousness and was dragged back to the dugout. The pitch had split my batting helmet.

Does a history of head injuries increase the chances of developing Alzheimer's? The evidence is still speculative, but it is known that head injuries can worsen the symptoms of Alzheimer's and hasten their onset, which brings me to a visit I had with my mother one January a couple years after I sobered up and started at *Guideposts*.

I was in the Detroit area for a story and planned to spend the night with my mother. I got to her house on Pebbleshire—this was before Joe and Toni moved her next door to them—at dinnertime and let myself in. Mom was setting the table. When she turned to hug me, I barely recognized her. The right side of her forehead was grossly swollen and deformed. There was a scabbed over cut that probably could have used a stitch or two. Her left eye was bruised black and vivid purple, the discoloration spreading over her cheekbone and turning a sickly green.

"Mom, what happened?"

"It looks worse than it is." Denial, the opening gambit.

"It looks awful. Are you all right?"

"I'm fine. Here, sit down. I made dinner."

I don't remember what she made. As I've said, Mom was an indifferent cook at best, not because she couldn't cook but because she wasn't that interested in it. To her, frozen dinners had been manna from heaven back in the '60s. A decade later she thought the girls I brought home from college in prairie skirts who wanted to make bread from scratch were loony.

"Don't change the subject. What happened to you?"

It turns out she was shoveling snow a few nights earlier, something most of us agree a seventy-something woman living alone shouldn't be doing. But that was my mother. At the slightest hint of snow—and in Michigan that's half the year—she'd be out with her shovel and no gloves taking care of business, day or night.

"I guess I slipped on some ice."

For a moment it looked like that was all the information I was going to elicit from this conversation as she steeped her tea bag a little longer than necessary and avoided eye contact.

"And?"

"I think I smacked my head on the bumper of the car."

She was still driving my dad's old Monte Carlo with the heavy stainless-steel bumper. Ow.

"You think? Did you lose consciousness?"

"I don't remember," she said, irritation creeping into her voice. She hated to be interrogated.

"You could have frozen to death."

"I was a little dizzy is all. I had a slight headache for a while."

"Did you take something for it?"

"Of course not."

"Did you call someone?"

"Don't be silly."

I stared at her. She could have been Quasimodo's twin sister her face was so deformed. And now I noticed a little cut and swelling on her lip.

"Mom, you really did a face-plant."

"I'm all right."

"I'd be surprised if you were. You need to get checked out."

"What's the point? It's just a bump on the head. Let's just forget about it."

Ironically as it would turn out, that phrase "Let's just forget about it" was a favorite of Mom's and meant that a conversation was over, done, the subject changed.

My entreaties for her to see a doctor were futile, as I should have known they would be. She didn't believe in doctors or think much of them, didn't take medication, not even vitamins until late in life, and it is still a mystery how that came about or who convinced her. Probably someone at church. The only conceivable reason to go to the hospital was to give birth, and I suspect she would have done that at home if she could. Maybe it was all the time she spent in doctors' offices with me as a severely asthmatic child, riding trollies to specialists all over Philadelphia, or all the health woes my father endured and doctors he saw that completely turned her off to modern medicine. We used to whisper that she was a secret Christian Scientist. I doubt she ever had a mammogram or a Pap smear. She also "never got sick" and even when she did, which was indeed rare, she never admitted it. Her cure for the common cold was to scrub the kitchen floor. And pray for others who were sick.

Looking back, I wonder if that head injury helped bring on the more overt symptoms of dementia that were soon to appear. It didn't cause her Alzheimer's. Yet it was an early indication, a warning, one of many early signs we should have paid more attention to, things we were too willing to write off as Mom's quirks. She was always a little flighty, a multitasker before they coined that term. She'd make breakfast while finishing a crossword puzzle and listening to the news and talking to one of us. No wonder she lost track of stuff from time to time. Age, we figured, only amplified the tendency.

• • •

IN THE SPRING OF THAT YEAR, I VISITED again while I was in town on some business or other. We had dinner with no mention of her fall. I had the urge to ask if she remembered it but didn't. It would have made her angry either because she couldn't remember or had completely repressed the episode. In any case, I didn't want to ruin the evening. The Tigers were playing an early season game and we loved watching together.

As was my wont, I went for a long walk after dinner, strolling the streets of Balmoral Orchards, where I used to ride my bike endlessly as a kid, wondering who still lived in their houses, who went crazy with the house paint, whose home looked down at the heels or empty, who might have died. I found myself at a small manmade lake at the center of the subdivision, an attempt at a touch of nature in a cookie-cutter neighborhood carved out of a former apple orchard. It was the lake where my twelve-year-old brother's body was found floating and bloated on an April day not unlike this, a month after he mysteriously disappeared some twenty years earlier.

There was never agreement on how his body got there, since shortly after his disappearance the Oakland County Sheriff declared if there was one place Bobby would not be found it was in that lake, which was covered by several feet of ice the day he disappeared and searched by men on horseback the next day. Bobby weighed maybe 100 pounds. And yet that lake is where they found him and no one could ever really explain it. There was a fight over closing the case and the chief investigator quit in protest.

As I turned and headed back, I spotted a still figure on the other side of the lake, gazing out over the water. Closer, I recognized Mom.

"What are you doing out here?"

She seemed startled. Then she said, "I was looking for you. I thought you were lost."

It didn't make any sense. I wasn't going to get lost, and she had never done this before. I knew this geography better than any place on earth. Despite its puffed up Anglophilic name, Balmoral Orchards was of modest size with a pretty straightforward street grid. We started walking. Mom suddenly veered down a street, going away from her house.

"Hey, Mom, we're going this way."

She paused. "Oh," she eventually said, "I thought you might still want to keep walking."

I steered her in the right direction, and we talked about the Tigers all the way down Pebbleshire. She told me they were winning, she thought, 4–1 over the White Sox. When we got home, I noticed that actually there was no score yet and they were playing the Twins.

How easy it would have been to correct Mom about the game. I wanted to. But doing so might have only upset her. She was having a hard enough time. I wasn't going to help the situation by telling her she was wrong about something.

As for the effects of alcoholism and head injuries on the development of Alzheimer's, that is a question I would continue to pursue.

• • •

Here are three things I learned dealing with my mother in the early stages of dementia—things you might benefit from if your loved one is in the early stages of the disease:

- **Don't push too hard.** Ask your questions gently and if the answer you get sounds off, don't push it or argue. Move on to another topic.

- **Listen. Carefully.** You can learn a lot about how your loved one's mind is processing information by simply letting them talk and not interrupting.

- **Make notes about your conversation afterwards.** You can refer back to them later to see if and how your loved one's condition has changed.

CHAPTER SIX

THE NATURE OF MIRACLES

A few weeks after my visit with the neurologist, Dr. Salinas, and after several days haggling with my insurance company over who would pay for it, I showed up for the MRI of my brain that the doctor had ordered. It was at an NYU-affiliated facility near Stuyvesant Park, close to where Julee and I had our first apartment.

Thinking about my mother's head injury—and my own—made getting the test seem like something I shouldn't put off, even with Covid surging again.

About 40 million MRI scans are conducted annually in the U.S., so I can safely assume that many of you have undergone the test and with varying degrees of trepidation. Especially for the claustrophobic. Fortunately, this was not my first time in the tube. I had to have an MRI prior to left hip replacement surgery, after burning out the joint doing indoor cycling classes practically every day for more than twenty years. (No, nothing compulsive about me!)

I also had some other kind of scan of my brain following yet another concussion I sustained going back for a deep fly ball playing center field for the *Guideposts* softball team and falling hard in the outfield. I want you know that I held onto the ball for the out, though I have little recollection of playing the rest of the game and after the last out had to inquire who won. The next day my doctor diagnosed retrograde amnesia due to mild concussion and sent me to a facility that scanned my brain using something that looked like an old-fashioned salon hair dryer, just to make sure there wasn't a bleed.

This would be my first time in the tube for a full brain scan, which would take about forty minutes. I was a little nervous, so I decided to use some of that energy by walking to the appointment, about forty-five blocks. Besides, taxis and mass transit were still a bit iffy due to the coronavirus. It was a humid late April afternoon. A chalky sky hovered low over the city and many pedestrians were prematurely wearing shorts and tank tops, jumping the gun on summer. Others were still entombed in Michelin Man puffer-style coats. It had been a long cold Covid winter. Some people dress for the weather and some people dress for the calendar I suppose.

On the way across town, it struck me that the inventor of the MRI, Dr. Raymond Damadian, once told his personal story in *Guideposts*. He was a man of both science and faith, and at a crucial moment in the development of the first MRI, it was faith that came to the rescue of science.

Dr. Damadian was not raised with faith but his college sweetheart and future wife, Donna, took him to a Billy Graham crusade, where he committed himself to a relationship with the Lord and vowed to go wherever He led. It interested me that after his undergraduate career majoring in mathematics at the University of Wisconsin he studied violin at Juilliard and played Junior Davis Cup Tennis prior to completing his medical degree at the Albert Einstein College of Medicine in New York. A true Renaissance man. I try not to compare myself.

Where the Lord led Dr. Damadian was research science, and early on he envisioned a new imaging technology that would be far more effective than X-rays in providing a detailed reading of the inner workings of the body. It would be like going from grainy black-and-white photography to 3D Technicolor.

There were many setbacks on the road to the first MRI as Dr. Damadian grew more obsessed with perfecting his invention. He believed it would be a game changer in diagnostic medicine and save countless lives with early detection of disease. In his fervor to invent the MRI he drifted from his church and his faith, all his energy going into the quest. Not that he became an unbeliever; he merely forgot to believe.

Years of frustration followed. Finally, he reached the point where failure seemed imminent. He confided his fears to Donna and her mother. "Don't worry," they said, "we are praying for you. Remember that."

The struggle continued and so did the prayers, and at last Dr. Damadian and his team succeeded in testing the first functional MRI machine, called an NMR scanner at the time.

Sharing his excitement with his family Dr. Damadian finally understood that God's hand had been on the project the whole time through the intercessory prayers of his wife, mother-in-law, and many others they had enlisted. Dr. Damadian concluded his *Guideposts* story by stating, "The thrill of science is the search to understand a small corner of God's grand design, and to lay the glory for such discoveries at the Grand Designer's feet."

• • •

As I strode across town, the odd recollection of that story seemed like a nudge from above, assurance that I had nothing to worry about, at least as far as the test went. By more than mere chance both my neurologist and the genius who invented the MRI machine had shared their stories in *Guideposts*. That did not seem like an accident. The results were another thing. Standing before the facility, I made a quick iPhone video to post on Guideposts.org and said a prayer for calm. I tried to envision myself relaxed and peaceful for the duration of the procedure.

I was grateful I didn't have to wait long for my turn in the machine. I was surprised by how little prep there was. All I was asked to do was exchange my standard-issue Covid surgical mask for one that didn't have a metal nosepiece.

"The metal can interfere with the machine," the technician explained. I certainly didn't want to be responsible for breaking one of Dr. Damadian's machines. I remember what happened once when I put some frozen mac and cheese in an aluminum container in my microwave.

"Should I remove my shoes?" I asked, for no particular reason at all.

He looked at me quizzically. "No," he said. "Why would you do that? This is a study of your brain. Keep your shoes on."

Maybe I was just nervous.

He slipped a giant protective set of headphones over my ears, made a few adjustments, then hit a button that slid the table I was lying faceup on into the machine.

Thank God for the protective headphones. The sounds the machine was making would have otherwise been deafening. As it was, the clanging was unnerving. I closed my eyes and wondered what parts of my brain were being probed. Was this even wise?

I thought back to Dr. Damadian's story, how this machine was born of faith as much as technology. I tried to think of tiny angels fluttering through my brain. looking for damaged neurons and synapses and wondered if they would have seen the same things in my mother's brain, those synaptic gaps and clusters of troublesome proteins. What is a brain after all but three pounds of gelatinous fat, water, protein, carbohydrates, and salts? It is a miracle that that mush can accomplish so much, from running the complexities of our metabolism and organ systems, to discovering relativity and the structure of DNA, to painting the ceiling of the Sistine Chapel. It is that mush that rules the world.

Angels or not, they were making an awful racket between my ears and the headphones were uncomfortable.

The MRI was over sooner than I expected, and I didn't know if that was a good thing or not. "You see anything in there?" I asked the technician. He smiled. "You know I can't comment. You'll get a full report from a radiologist in a day or two. Log into your chart. It should be there."

"Thanks."

"You do have a brain, if that helps."

"It might put some people at ease."

●   ●   ●

OUTSIDE I MADE ANOTHER QUICK VIDEO FOR THE website, my ears still ringing from the infernal bonging of the MRI. I wasn't planning on returning to the Berkshires until later in the week, so I wandered over to lovely little Stuyvesant Square, a stone's throw from our first apartment, a tiny sublet walk-up Julee and I inhabited our first year together. We used to bring Rudy, the cocker spaniel who introduced us, here. The park was first developed by the great-great-grandson of Peter Stuyvesant, his celebrated relative having been known for his famous peg leg and his leadership of the colony of New Netherland, whose capital New Amsterdam would eventually become New York after the English moved in and more or less stole it.

The land for the park was carved out of the Stuyvesant farm. There is a magnificent 200-year-old English elm towering above the western entrance and a lovely central fountain and a statue of Old Peg Leg himself, as well as one of the Czech Romantic composer Antonin Dvorak, who lived nearby after settling in America in the late nineteenth century. The park affords a good view of historic St. George's Episcopal Church, right around the corner from the Friends Meeting House and Seminary. (And you thought Manhattan was where the godless ran wild. You can scarcely walk a block without encountering a church, synagogue, or mosque, most of which have an AA meeting going on in the basement.)

Back in the nasty '70s you might have been right about the city's seedy decline. After dark, Stuyvesant Square was no place to be, a dangerous and notorious locale for all sorts of low assignations and hookups. You could barely walk ten feet without tripping over a used hypodermic.

Fortunately, the park enjoyed a comeback in the '80s, shortly before Julee and I moved there, and I have fond memories of it and still visit whenever I get the opportunity. My mother loved this park when she came to visit, and we would walk Rudy there in the morning while drinking our coffee. On the western edge there is a former lying-in maternity hospital, build in 1902, where women spent a month(!) convalescing from childbirth. It was converted into luxury condos around the time Julee and I arrived and renamed Rutherford Place.

We used to love to go look at apartments there, though we could not have even afforded a closet in one of those über-posh units. It was exciting to dream, though, and the sales agents were very indulgent since we lived across the street, and they loved Rudy. The big news was that David Byrne was buying in the building. I don't know if he ever did and today Rutherford Place contains mostly medical offices and suites as well as some luxe apartments.

I took a seat on a bench in view of the fountain and watched the arcing sprays of water, imagining they formed angel wings like the ones I pictured infiltrating my brain, but on a grander scale. Maybe a few of you don't believe angels exist at all or adhere to strict Biblical visages of mighty masculine warriors of the firmament who would be unlikely to dance on the head of a pin. Then there are the fearsome gargoyle-like entities described in Ezekiel. Or perhaps you imagine two men in suits and ties, their wings tucked inside their jackets.

For thirty years our sister publication *Angels on Earth* magazine has told true personal stories of people's encounters with angels. The editors of the magazine interpret these messengers as something more than just full-fledged winged seraphs who swoop to the rescue like heavenly superheroes. Angels can come in all shapes and sizes. Sometimes an angel is a breath of wind or a strain of music at just the right moment, or a feeling that has been inexplicably instilled in you and lifts you up as if on the wings of...well, you get it. An angel can also be, and frequently is, another human being who acts in an angelic way. We all have those angels in our lives. Where would we be without them?

Through the years the magazine—and there is no other magazine like it—has told many stories of angels who give comfort and aid to those afflicted by Alzheimer's and their families—angels of mercy, angels of reassurance, angels who lend strength, angels of solace. I would like to tell one of my favorite's here.

• • •

IN THE FOOTHILLS OF THE PYRENEES IN SOUTHWESTERN France, lies the town of Lourdes, one of the most popular pilgrimage destinations in the world for the purported healing properties of the waters there. According to a young Catholic girl named Bernadette, on the evening of February 11, 1858, the Virgin Mary appeared to her in a grotto, or small cave, imparted church doctrine to her, and subsequently instructed her to dig in the ground at a specific spot and drink from the water of a spring that bubbled up.

In the years since, millions of ailing pilgrims have sought the healing powers the waters are said to possess and thousands of cures have been reported, though less than a hundred have been scientifically validated and accepted by the Catholic Church. More important than the miraculous cures themselves, I think, is that these are the waters of hope, the belief that healing can be spiritual as well as physical. Perhaps that is the greatest miracle of Lourdes, the miracle of hope through the power of belief.

continued on p. 133

• • •

TIM YOUNG OF Edina, Minnesota, had pilgrimaged twice to Lourdes to seek relief from diabetes, and while his condition did not improve significantly, the visits deepened his faith, his sense of hope that he was cared for by a loving, healing God.

He didn't think a visit to Lourdes would cure his lifelong friend, Walter, of Alzheimer's, but he wanted Walter to experience the holiness of Lourdes before it was too late. Tim himself grew convinced Lourdes was what some people call a thin place, where the veil between the earthly and the spiritual realms is diaphanous.

Walter's dementia, though worsening, was still not yet so debilitating that it prevented him from traveling. Tim and Walter had known each other since childhood, and how much longer Walter would know Tim was in doubt.

All his life Tim had looked up to Walter, had turned to him for advice and support. Walter had always been there for Tim. Now Tim needed to be there for Walter. He assured Walter's wife, Carol, that he would take good care of him.

It was not as easy as Tim expected. On the flight over Walter kept trying to light up a cigarette. Tim patiently explained to the flight crew his friend's dementia, but after the third and fourth attempt Tim had to confiscate Walter's cigarettes and lighter.

At busy Charles de Gaulle Airport in Paris, Walter tried to use the ladies' room instead of the men's until Tim diverted him at the last second. He would introduce himself to random strangers for no reason. Getting him to say the name of their destination correctly was nearly impossible. Tim himself could hardly say Lourdes with the proper French pronunciation but his efforts to teach Walter were utterly futile.

Arriving in Lourdes at last, the two men dropped their bags at their hotel and went to visit the famous grotto and springs, crowded with visitors from around the world. On the way Walter asked where they were going.

"To the shrine at Lourdes, remember?"

Walter just stared blankly.

At first Tim wasn't sure Walter felt the holiness of the place the way he did, his soul stirred by the sacred waters and the prayers of the faithful. He prayed Walter would be moved. Then he noticed Walter staring at the beautiful statue of Mary inside the grotto, transfixed, focused in a way he hadn't been all during the long trip from Minnesota.

They walked back to the hotel in silence. A light spring rain had started to fall, and Tim tried to shield Walter with his umbrella. Walter didn't seem to notice. At the hotel Walter promptly planted himself on a couch in the lobby and said, "I'm hungry!" Of course. It was nearly past dinnertime and they'd barely eaten all day.

"Okay, you stay right here, Walter. I'll be back."

Tim dashed up to their room to check in with Carol before she retired for the night and let her know they'd made it to Lourdes safely and Walter was doing okay. He didn't mention him trying to smoke cigarettes on the airliner.

"Where's Walter now?" she asked.

"I told him to wait for me in the lobby."

"Not a good idea, Tim."

Tim hung up and rushed back down. Carol had been right. Walter was nowhere to be seen. *I should never have left him*, Tim thought. He could have kicked himself. He checked the restaurant. No Walter. He looked in the gift shop, filled with knickknacks of the shrine, and the lounge. Nobody had seen anyone matching Walter's description, which was standard-issue American tourist.

Tim ran to the main entrance and peered out the doors. The rain was coming down hard now and he could barely see anything in the dim streetlights. He quickly found the hotel's manager, Jean-Michel, in his office and explained the situation, trying to keep the panic out of his voice.

"Do not worry, monsieur," the manager said. "We will find your friend. He can't have wandered far."

Jean-Michel gathered his staff in the lobby and organized a search. They covered the hotel from top to bottom, checking elevators, stairwells, empty rooms, utility closets, every place they could think of. Still no Walter. Tim was in anguish. There was no telling what could happen to a man in Walter's condition in a strange town in a foreign country.

"The police will locate him," Jean-Michel said and dialed the precinct. Meanwhile, Tim was on edge. He ran back to his room, considered calling Carol but thought better of it, then grabbed his umbrella and headed out into the night of an unfamiliar city in search of his friend. He'd let Walter down after a lifetime of

Walter standing by him. He had to find him and prayed for God's guidance and protection of his friend in between bouts of excoriating himself for being so foolish.

Throughout the night Tim crisscrossed the streets, trying to keep his bearings. He was soaked to the bone and his shoes were so waterlogged that they squeaked as he walked. He returned to the grotto hoping Walter might have been drawn there and was met with darkness and silence and despair.

Around midnight the rain ended, and a sharp wind rose. As he crossed the deserted town square the moon appeared from behind the scudding clouds. Tim gazed up at a church steeple outlined against the night sky. He prayed again for Walter's protection. *Begged* would be a better word for it.

He got back to the hotel just before dawn and asked the night clerk, "Any sign of my friend?"

"Non, monsieur."

He took a hot shower and changed into dry clothes. He thought about calling Carol but decided to wait until he heard from the police.

Jean-Michel met him in the lobby and informed him that the police had turned up nothing. He patted Tim on the shoulder and said, "Tell you what. Let's go in my car and drive the town. We're bound to see your friend in the daylight."

"Thank you."

The streets were crowded with tourists, all seemingly dressed like Walter. Jean-Michel stopped at shops and cafés to inquire about a missing American who might be acting strangely. Still there was no sign of Walter. As they drove back to the hotel Jean-Michel turned and said with all earnestness, "My friend, Lourdes is a town of angels. They watch over us and I am sure they are watching over your friend. Here, angels are everywhere. That's why people come."

Tim hoped and prayed the manager was right. Poor Walter!

They returned to the hotel to find a police car parked in front. Tim rushed into the lobby. There was a knot of policemen standing around Walter, who was sitting in the exact spot on the couch where Tim had left him thirty-six hours earlier. Tim was so weak with relief and gratitude he nearly collapsed.

"Walter, where have you been?"

Walter looked at him blankly. "When?" he finally said.

"Where did they find him?" Tim asked Jean-Michel, who translated for the police.

"They say he just appeared at the precinct. No one knows how he got there."

Jean-Michel brought a wonderfully prepared French meal up to Walter and Tim's room. Tim's questions only confused Walter so he stopped asking about where his friend had been. Even stranger, Walter was not the least bit hungry, even though he almost certainly went all night without eating. Stranger still, Walter's clothes and shoes were bone-dry even after a night out in the rain. How could that be?

Tim remembered what Jean-Michel said about angels and how Tim himself believed Lourdes to be a thin place. It was clear to him now that his friend had somehow been watched over and protected in this place of hope and spiritual healing.

One other thing. On the flight back to the States Walter was calm. No ill-advised attempts at cigarette smoking. No misadventures in the restrooms. Most interesting of all was whenever Tim said the word *Lourdes* in his upper Midwest accent, Walter would correct him, using the perfect French pronunciation. *Who,* Tim couldn't help wondering, *taught him that?*

As I sat on the bench in Stuyvesant Park gazing at the fountain I thought about the nature of miracles. Miracles of science, like the MRI machine I'd just spent some time in. The miracle of a lost man being looked over by angels. The miracle of a tree that's grown for over 200 years. All around us are miracles if we merely open our eyes to God's grace and glory. I will end here with the words of St. Augustine.

"Miracles are not in contradiction to nature. They are only in contradiction with what we know of nature."

CHAPTER SEVEN

A SLOWLY LENGTHENING SHADOW

Alzheimer's is like a slowly lengthening shadow that casts itself over the life of the sufferer and her family. Little slips become larger issues. Things that in our seemingly infinite capacity for denial we desperately try to ignore or explain away or control. There seems to be one inevitable turning point all families reach: having to take away driving privileges, literally taking away the keys. The keys to freedom and mobility, as if the disease has finally taken you prisoner.

I've heard of families where this is an easy, natural transition. But that is rare. For the most part this is a kind of moment of truth.

Maybe that's because we are such a mobile, automotive-centric culture, especially in a city like Detroit and its suburbs, built on the internal combustion engine, where public transit is practically a dirty word.

After Toni and Joe moved Mom into the house next door to them, Toni said Mom was in and out of that driveway constantly, always coming and going—to church, the grocery store, TJ Maxx, her volunteer shifts at The Resource Center. "She is always going in and out of that driveway," Toni said. And I had the uneasy feeling she didn't always know where she was going or why. But that was Mom, always on the move, *having* to keep moving, one foot on the brake and one foot on the accelerator, so the car proceeded down the road like a gazelle.

• • •

MOM DIDN'T LEARN TO DRIVE UNTIL SHE WAS well into her forties, during our last years in Philly. My father was, well, old school about women driving, to put it kindly. And back in Philly public transit was plentiful. We didn't live in a suburb, we lived in a neighborhood. Most everything you needed was in walking or trolley car distance. If there were any more distant parts of the city Mom yearned to visit, Dad would be happy to drive her. In fact, he loved driving. So, we were a one-car family.

Until Mom finally broke through. She'd lobbied hard for a driver's license and a car for a long time. Her two sisters, Cass and Marion, drove cars (Cass drove a Welcome Wagon in Paoli out on the Main Line). Joe and Mary Lou would soon be old enough to drive. Then there were Bobby and me, who needed to be carted around. It was just too much without a car. Knowing how strong-willed and independent she was, it's hard to imagine why it took her so many years to get my father to relent. She must have made his life very difficult. In the end, though, she won, and Dad signed her up for driving lessons…and himself up for an ulcer.

I'd go with her in the evenings to a driving school where they started you out on a very primitive driving simulator. Looking back, I can't imagine anyone learning to operate a motor vehicle that way. It was like something adapted from a carnival ride. I think it was more of a gimmick to drag out the classes before they put you in the real thing. It was fun for me, though. If there was a simulator not being used, I got to sit in it and mess around with the dashboard, great fun for a six-year-old already dreaming of his own license and all the places he would go.

So, Mom passed her driving test after the second try and Dad bought her a used, two-tone black and red Plymouth. I have no idea where he found this car. He liked sleek new cars like Pontiac Bonnevilles. We had a grape-green one he was incredibly proud of. I couldn't imagine why he would allow a bulbous heap like the Plymouth to be seen with it in the same driveway. It must have hurt.

On her very first time out on the road solo in the Plymouth she sideswiped a cop, and not before she got very far. It couldn't have been a more perfect realization of my father's darkest fears. Of course, that wasn't all. She proceeded to blame the cop for the accident—*he* wasn't watching where he was going—and my mother was not one to quit on an argument. Fortunately, my father happened by and kept her from being put in handcuffs. On that inaugural journey Mom got her first ticket and Dad his first repair bill. It escapes me now where Mom was going that day and I have a feeling she was just driving to get a feel for the freedom of it, because that's what driving gave her right in the middle of her life: independence.

• • •

DECADES LATER IN MICHIGAN THE PROSPECT OF DEPRIVING her of that hard-won independence was gut-wrenching. I couldn't think about it without every cell in my body cringing. I didn't want to think about it. Yet there had just been too many incidents. Twice she crashed through the back of the garage (she blamed the car). Another sideswiping in Birmingham that she was evidently oblivious to until a cop caught up to her and, yes, found himself in a fierce argument about how he was mistaken and needed to stop wasting time and go find the real culprit.

How we kids—a social worker, a civil litigator married to another civil litigator, and me, for what my judgments are worth—could have let her menace the highways and byways for so long and put herself and other people in danger is baffling and uncharacteristically irre-sponsible. We knew better.

Joe had already taken over her finances, balancing her checkbook and keeping her bills straight, especially all the donations she was making to foreign missionaries. Mom did not have her own bank account until her late fifties. It was another pseudo-Victorian quirk of my father's. Then one day she demanded to have her own savings account (the motive, I suspect, being that I was just starting college and she wanted to be able to surreptitiously slip me cash). She prevailed rather quickly this time and she and Dad went to the Detroit Bank and Trust branch in nearby Franklin and opened an account, whereupon he took the passbook and said, "So, anytime you need to take out some money just ask me for the passbook."

That item never reached his pocket. I'm told her arm shot out like a striking cobra and snatched it from his hand.

Nevertheless, Dad still paid the bills until he died a few years before Mom's symptoms emerged and she took them over. By the time Joe got involved the bill keeping had deteriorated to the point where we could have used a forensic audit to straighten things out.

Taking away the car keys was a monumental step beyond this. It meant getting rid of all the denial and guilt and fear and doing something you know is right even if you hate yourself for doing it. And I hated myself when I thought about how hard she'd fought for those keys, that freedom, just to have it snatched away by her kids, cruelly and arbitrarily to her mind.

You start out life with your parents making decisions for you and suddenly, years later, you find yourself making decisions for them. It feels wrong. It feels taboo, Alzheimer's or no Alzheimer's, and I tried to blame the disease and not my mom. Yet the prospect filled me with dread because I knew exactly how she would react. I was too much like her not to know, not to feel already what she was going to feel. I wanted to pray that this bitter cup be passed from me, to not drink of this sadness.

I remember her once suddenly saying to me about her older sister, "You know, they won't let Marion drive anymore." The statement came from nowhere, which meant it came from somewhere deep and hidden, something she'd been thinking about until the words just forced themselves out. I didn't know what to say in response except that one day it might be her. I was sorry the second I said it. My mom acted as if she didn't hear me. Didn't want to hear me.

Joe, Mary Lou, and I made a plan. I would fly out for one of my periodic visits. Julee and Toni wisely demurred. They thought this was one thing the children themselves alone had to undertake. They didn't want Mom to feel ganged up on.

She did anyway.

•   •   •

I THINK SHE KNEW IT WAS COMING. WE sat around her kitchen table and laid out the case. She'd had accidents. She'd lost her car in a parking lot several times and then lost her way coming home. We didn't say she had classic Alzheimer's symptoms. We didn't go there. We said it wasn't safe for her to drive anymore and didn't go any deeper. This was hard enough without opening other, more dreadful doors. *Mom, you have an irreversible, untreatable terminal brain disease just like your sisters and we've got to get you off the road.* And so we simply said please if we could just have the keys to the car, we'll help you with other arrangements for getting around.

"You're the ones who are crazy," she said.

So much for that.

"No one said anything about being crazy, Mom," Mary Lou said.

"I haven't lost my mind!"

"Nobody's saying that," I said. It struck me that Alzheimer's as a condition, as an organic disease of the brain with a distinct set of pathologies, was not how my mother's generation necessarily interpreted it. They saw it more as a form of madness, something darker, something akin to a curse or a sin, or that age-old enfeeblement, senility. Maybe we should have had a frank medical discussion first. Now

I wish we had, no matter how heartbreaking that would have been. Brought a doctor in. Maybe a priest.

"You're not taking my car. I need my car. How will I get anywhere? Who are you to tell me I can't drive!"

She knew this had happened to Cass and her Welcome Wagon gig, and to Marion, of course, and to others she knew from St. Owen's. Now this fate had closed in on her and she wasn't having it.

"You're not taking my car!" she said, jumping up from the table and pacing around the kitchen. Nobody paced like Estelle Grinnan, except maybe me.

"There's nothing wrong with my driving. Other people are bad drivers."

"Mom, let us have the keys," Joe said.

She had started to cry, tears of confusion and anger and defiance. She was backed up against the sink like a cornered animal, holding her bag. The suncatcher behind her said, "Prayer changes everything." Could it? Could it change this, Lord, this depth of awfulness and betrayal I felt? Betrayal.

After she lost Bobby, nobody would have blamed her if she never let me out of her sight, especially with the mystery surrounding his disappearance that cold winter day, a mystery that left the deepest scars a mother can sustain. Who could have blamed her for becoming neurotically overprotective, of strangling me with her apron strings? What could possibly destroy one's sense of security in this world more than a child who disappears into thin air and a month later turns up dead with more questions than answers?

But she didn't. She knew I needed my independence because she knew how much I was like her. That I needed that air to breathe, to become the person she knew I was meant to be. I enjoyed the kind of freedom most kids today couldn't conceive of. Maybe too much freedom at times, freedom to run away from things I couldn't face. Freedom to find things I shouldn't have found.

Now I was taking her freedom, wresting her independence away, and it felt like a primal betrayal.

Except she wouldn't give us the keys. She absolutely refused to surrender them and none of us had the moxie to physically tear her bag from her hands and seize them. It ended up a standoff and the three of us children beat a retreat to Joe's house to consider our next steps. A little mindless voice in my head said, "Good for her."

• • •

I WAS STAYING AT MOM'S BUT BY THE time I got back she'd already gone to bed, which was a little out of the ordinary since she had become kind of a night bird and usually we'd stay up late talking politics or sports. I retired to the guest room and slumped on the bed, defeated and exhausted. With my toe I pulled my carry-on over to me, unzipped the main compartment, and out rolled two cans of my now-warm beer.

Two sixteen-ounce Ballantine beers, to be exact. How had they gotten there?

I stared at them as if they were apparitions. Of course, I'd packed them, though I didn't remember doing it. That will sound strange to a non-dipsomaniac, but these things happen to alcoholics.

The fact was, I had recently been drinking again secretly, alone, in relatively small amounts, after nearly six years of sobriety. Six years. I can't explain it other than saying alcoholics drink, and the drink is always waiting. I remember the absurd circumstances of my first drink after all those years of abstinence and meetings.

Julee had stepped in to take over singer Cindy Wilson's role in The B-52s rock band while Cindy started a family, and they were kicking off a summer tour with an appearance on *The Tonight Show* in Los Angeles. Do you realize how many midwestern kids like Julee dream of that? *The Tonight Show?*

A few hours before the show aired in New York I was walking our cocker spaniel, Sally Browne, past a store on Third Avenue when I saw a cooler inside packed with exotic beers. One called Anchor Steam caught my eye. I'd never had the pleasure. Why shouldn't a man be able to enjoy a beer while watching his wife perform on *The Tonight Show*? So, Sally and I went in and almost as if in a kind of fugue state, I purchased two bottles of Anchor Steam, more shocked at how much beer prices had risen than by the fatal mistake I was making.

The beers sat peacefully in the fridge for the hours leading up to the show. I popped the first one as the theme music came on and Jay Leno launched into his monologue. The beer had a slightly sour aftertaste, though I never drank for the taste. I opened the second one for the B's performance, sipping it through the interview afterwards. When they cut to commercial, I dumped the rest down the kitchen drain. There. No need to finish it. I had a grip on this.

It had been a long time since I had alcohol in my system, but I slept well. The morning was bright and summery. I wasn't hung over but there was a slight glow to everything as I walked to work, like a corona effect. Clearly something had changed.

Now I was staring at those two Ballantines. My secret drinking had worsened, no longer confined to when Julee was touring. I brought these beers with me because I knew I would need them to quell the anxiety and guilt. I promised that these would be the last, but I always said that.

• • •

IT WASN'T LONG AFTER OUR CONFRONTATION WITH HER that Mom was finally taken off the road. Toni noticed some new dents on her car. Mom claimed a truck drove into her driveway and caused the damage, then drove away. This, of course, made no sense but Mom was still given to confabulation rather than admitting she didn't remember. Toni checked around with the police and discovered that you could anonymously report a dangerous driver and have them called in for retesting. She followed through and Mom got a letter requesting she take such an exam. Joe drove her in her car, Mom failed the test miserably, and her license, which she turned over before the test, was invalidated. Joe drove her home and kept the keys, later moving her car and keeping it in a parking structure at his office in case Mom remembered where she kept her spare set.

Back in New York I met these developments with considerable relief. We had waited too long to act and I could only thank the Lord that my mother hadn't caused a serious accident or injury. In fact, I think God and his angels kept watch over her on the road. That and St. Christopher, whose dashboard statuette always rode with her, despite his demotion by the Vatican. Mom was an obedient Catholic, but she had her limits.

You will not be surprised to learn that my periodic drinking did not stop that night in Michigan. Stopping and starting drinking, especially for an alcoholic who has experienced some years of recovery, is incredibly stressful, like walking a tightrope with your eyes closed and praying you don't fall into the abyss. It's much easier to just get drunk all the time and not keep it secret.

There is a saying in AA that we are only as sick as our secrets. I was getting sicker and sicker, drinking whenever the opportunity arose, which generally came while Julee was touring. Her absence certainly wasn't the reason for my drinking; it only provided the opportunity. You can't thwart an alcoholic determined to drink from drinking. I always drank alone at home after work and on weekends. And woke up every morning in a state of terror that only abated with that first drink in the evening. I was increasingly taking time off from work and wondering how I would explain to Julee what happened to all that vacation time.

I got away with it at first. At least I thought I did. I held on to my job and paid the rent and managed to take care of our two dogs,

Sally and our young Lab, Marty. I say I drank alone. That's not true. I drank with the knowledge of my own disease. That knowledge was as real as a physical presence, a relentless realization that I was reversing years of growth and spiritual development and trashing my relationship with God, from whom I could hide nothing.

I prayed to stop drinking even though I knew I wouldn't. Those prayers were a lie. I lied to God, which is pretty far down the path to hell, at least metaphysically. That was the worst of it all—not that I was drinking but that I was being dishonest with my life. The lies will kill you; alcohol is just the manner of death.

It all came crashing down like I knew it would. Julee returned from L.A. one evening to find me passed out on the couch, bottles everywhere, the dogs hysterical, the apartment a mess, my own personal crime scene.

Had I not been so intoxicated I would have known she was coming home, but in the preceding days I'd more or less lost control and lost track of time. The first thing she did was run the dogs out for a quick walk. Then she got on the phone.

Julee loved me very much, but she grew up in a family where alcohol had been a problem and she wasn't about to let it become one in ours. "You can't stay here like this, Edward. I can't let you out on your own and I'm not going to a hotel. I've been living in hotels and I want my home. You're going to a detox. You can come back in a few days when you've sobered up. I've called Michael to help me."

I tried to pull myself together while Julee threw a few of my things in a small bag. "I'm not angry with you," she said. "You just can't stay here like this." Something told me she was not entirely surprised by this turn of events.

Michael and Julee helped me downstairs and into a cab. "Where are we going?" I asked, wedged between them.

"St. Luke's Roosevelt Hospital," Julee said. "They have a unit."

"It's locked," Michael added with a twinge of mordancy. "You can leave if you want but I wouldn't advise it."

"Speaking as a lawyer, of course," I slurred at him.

He just laughed and rolled down the window.

We arrived in minutes and the next thing I knew I was being half-dragged down a long hallway with gruesome fluorescent lighting at the end of which were a set of red double doors. My wife had me by one arm and my friend by the other. As we neared the end I attempted some token resistance that Michael recognized immediately as a ruse and moved me along. An image of my mother resisting our efforts to get her car keys away from her blinked in my mind. Her defiance was so much more genuine than mine.

The red doors opened. Julee gave me a hard hug and Michael patted me on the back saying, "Get better." Then I was turned over to a large, older nurse whose eye shadow looked like the chalk used on a pool cue and whose lipstick was the color of dried blood. Or it might just have been the lighting.

• • •

DETOXES ARE NOT MEANT TO BE NICE PLACES, unless you check in to one of those posh country club facilities, and this was not that. Detoxes are not rehabs; they're medical landing pads where you're quickly taken off one substance by substituting another—methadone for heroin, Valium for alcohol, etc. Sadly, most are revolving doors for addicts and drunks.

I was very interested in getting my first dose of Valium to ward off the shakes and withdrawal angst but first there was a perfunctory intake process, then a talk with a doctor. I was already pacing when he came into my room and introduced himself. I don't recall his name, but he was younger than me. He took a quick medical history, did an even quicker exam, including a prostate palpation, which I thought was completely uncalled for, made me stick my tongue out to check for tremors, asked how much alcohol I drank, and sat silently for a good long time scribbling notes while I went silently crazy. At one point he let his gaze linger on me for a second or two as if it had just occurred to him that there was something out-of-place about me.

"I'm awfully shaky," I finally said. The drink had mostly worn off by now. My heart rate was rising, I could feel my pulse pounding in my ears, and I was clammy.

"I'll give you something for that." He closed his file on me, reached into the pocket of his white doctor's smock, and produced a single dose pill in a tiny blister pack.

"This is 10 milligrams of Valium."

"Oh, no, that won't do," I said.

"This should help you rest, Mr. Grinnan."

"Believe me, it won't."

"Let's try it first then talk about next steps."

"I should have an I.V."

"May I ask where you received your medical degree?"

He let that sink in for a minute then cracked a smile and got me some water to take the useless dose of Valium with.

"I'll be back," he said.

"I'm counting on it."

And he was, every time I hit my call button. I'm not sure how many milligrams of Valium he gave me before he gave up and I resigned myself to a sleepless forty-eight hours or so and the crippling anxiety and shakes that went with it.

The unit was relatively small but there was enough of a hallway for me to pass the hours pacing back and forth and praying for sleep to come, praying for relief from this dreadful metastasizing angst, making all sorts of quid-pro-quo deals with God. I listened to other patients snoring and muttering in their sleep. At one point they brought someone new in. I sensed a lot of restlessness. I was startled when a nurse came up from behind me.

"You really shouldn't be out of your room," she said, laying a warm, gentle hand on my shoulder.

"I can't sleep. I can't stay still. I'll go crazy."

"Let's get you back in bed and I'll have the doctor see you," she said. She was very kind. I let her bring me back to my room.

It was a new doctor, an even younger one. Shift change. He listened to my heart—nothing more intrusive—then reached into the pocket of his doctor's smock.

"We can try something different," he said softly, pulling out another blister pack containing two capsules the size of .45 caliber bullets. "I might get in trouble for this," he said. "This is a drug called chloral hydrate."

He held it out for me like a magician showing his trick deck of cards. I'm sure my eyes widened at this unknown philter; the name struck a vaguely familiar note.

"It's an old drug, more than a hundred years old actually, not used much anymore, but maybe it will help you sleep. People used it back in Victorian times. Very popular with the ladies."

Like the previous doctor, he got me some water and I swallowed the pills, not really believing dope from the nineteenth century was going to do anything. He stood and watched me for a moment, smiled quizzically, then turned to leave.

"Good night, Mr. Grinnan," he said, closing my door behind him.

My stomach was completely empty. Probably a couple days since I ate. I thought about sneaking out and pacing the hallway some more but when I got up, I felt the room tumble. I regained my balance. In fact, I felt definitely drowsy. Were these pills an answer to prayer? If so, God was good. I was sound asleep before I knew that answer.

In the years since that night, I've thought about that young doctor and his magic potion. The incident has never quite left me. I've read up on the drug. It is a drug from the nineteenth century, to be sure, much abused before the FDA came around, its use mostly banned today.

But was it real? Why would he risk his medical license by "getting into trouble" administering a dubious and archaic drug? And why would he admit that even if it were true? I've come to some conclusions about him. He was very clever indeed. He set me up beautifully with a couple of tricked-out placebos—sugar pills. He was a magician of sorts. He fooled my brain into believing it was drugged and sleepy and I slept. Quite a trick. An amazing trick, actually.

In writing this book I've come to believe that our minds are a labyrinth of memories and mirrors that can make its own reality, like me believing I had been sedated by a chemical substance when in reality I hadn't. Yet that belief was induced in me. My brain conformed to that inducement and believed it was reality. It's also what happens often in the later stages of Alzheimer's, I've learned. It's what happened to my mother and her friend Pat. That is a story that comes later.

●   ●   ●

I AWOKE THE NEXT MORNING TO A CLATTERING of a plastic food tray with plastic hospital food deposited on my bedside table by an orderly who left without a word. I felt a little more back on my rails thanks to those pills and the sleep they conferred.

I picked at the breakfast, wondering what to do with myself, then wandered out to the day room. The walls were drab and colorless, though there was evidence of an attempt to add some brightness and geometric designs, long faded. The air was stuffy and the general atmosphere desultory. There was a TV on that nobody was watching.

About a half dozen patients were there, a couple pacing and others resting or asleep at tables or in chairs. The Valium was still dulling my senses except for a growing sense of anxiety. How long would I be held? What about Julee? My work?

This train of thought was derailed by a woman who came right up to me.

"What are you doing here?" she demanded.

She was middle-aged and Hispanic with a Bronx accent and a Bronx proclivity for speaking her mind, apparently. I wasn't sure how to answer her question.

"I saw that coat you were wearing when they brought you in."

My coat. What did that mean? I could barely remember what I wore but I did own a relatively new suede coat, a bomber-style jacket. I wanted to tell her I bought it on sale but stopped myself, thank God.

"Ain't no one in here have a coat like that." Then her expression broke into one of bemusement. "Don't worry, no one gonna hurt you. This is a pretty safe place. It's the staff you gotta watch."

I scanned the room. There didn't seem to be any staff present. There was only one other white person, an older woman asleep in a chair who looked like she'd been rescued from the street. She wore hospital clothes but the rest, a young Black woman and several Black men of various ages, were all in street clothes, like me.

"I'm Della," my new friend said. "I'm a junkie. What about you?"

"Well, alcohol, I guess."

"You guess? You mean you're a drunk."

"Basically."

"I don't drink much. I got a bad stomach. Maybe smoke a little rock now and again. I been using heroin since I was a teenager. I got off a few times but always went back. That's just the way it is with junk. I hardly known anyone who beat it."

"I know people who've beat it," I said, thinking of some of the recovering addicts I'd met in the AA rooms.

"Not people like me."

Point taken.

"You got insurance?"

"Yes," I said.

"That's why they let you in here. They don't make enough money off us."

One of the young men sitting nearby laughed. "They make enough money off you, Del. You're a regular customer here."

"Shut up, Tony," Della said.

"Della runs out of cash to buy dope before the month runs out, she comes here."

"It ain't bad," she said. "They give you methadone, three squares, a bed. I just wait here till I get my check and then I'm out."

"The miracle of direct deposit!" Tony roared.

I must have look confused because Della said, "From the government. My check. When it comes in, I go out. Should be any day now. Lots of people do it."

Tony laughed and shook his head. "I wish it was that easy for me. I gotta go see the judge. They have a case on me. I gotta be clean."

"They test you?" Della asked.

"Oh yeah."

"You got a case?" Della asked me.

"Me? No. I have a wife who's awfully upset with me and a job I'm worried about."

Della gave me a look and a wry smile. "Don't you worry. They'll take care of you."

An unmistakable odor filled the room, the smell of reheated hospital food.

"Wonder what they're feeding us for lunch," she said.

"Same old thing, I suspect," Tony said.

"We'll get served last, as always." This last remark came from an older man who was using headphones and a battered Walkman. When he took off the headphones I could hear the tinny strains of a song I knew but couldn't put my finger on. Suddenly I knew it: "Thank You for Letting Me Be Myself, Again" by Sly Stone.

"I thought you couldn't bring anything in here like that," I said, wishing I had brought mine.

"You can't," Tony said. "Sometimes there's rules, sometimes there's not."

I strained to hear. I liked the song. The man noticed and turned up the volume. Sly's voice sounded even more compressed leaking through the headphones.

"You seen a counselor yet?" Della asked me.

"No," I said.

"You will. Probably this afternoon. I don't know who's on today. A couple of them are pretty nice but some of the others don't care. I can't blame them."

• • •

MY SUBSTANCE ABUSE COUNSELOR WAS CARL, WHO ROSE a few inches out of his chair, shook my hand, and sat back down in one swift movement. His desk was a mess, and he had a mesh-covered window that looked out on a brick wall about ten feet away.

"Have a seat," he said, rifling through a file, frowning, putting it aside and picking up another and turning it sideways so he could read the tab.

"Mr. Grinnan."

I nodded. He was about my age, presumably in recovery like most of them were, looked overworked but still willing to do his job, a job that can burn you out almost as badly as the addiction that motivated you to do something to help other addicts in the first place. He flipped through the pages and made a few notations. Checked off a box with a flourish.

"How are you feeling?"

"Better than I expected."

"Good."

"Still a little worried about withdrawal seizures."

"We're giving you something for that."

"I appreciate it."

"But just short term, to get you through the next couple days."

"Understood."

He inquired about my background—profession, education, family, home situation. General questions about my health, mental and physical. Probed my brother's death a little. They always do. I didn't say much. Wanted to know if I was suicidal.

"No more than usual," I said with a smile, then added, "Just trying to keep it light."

As a kid growing up in Michigan I played a lot of hockey, mostly as a goalie. The more personal Carl's questions got, the more I felt like I was back in the net on Wing Lake, blocking shots on goal. One question I batted out of the crease with my stick. Another hit my pad and I kicked it away. One I blocked with my shoulder and the question shot over the net. Another I gloved and tossed into the corner. I went to the ice on another, smothering it just before it could cross the goal line. A couple shots got through but most I artfully turned away.

"You've had a lot of sobriety over the past ten years or so since you first went to rehab."

"Right. Mostly I've been sober," I said. "Until recently."

"So, what made you pick it back up?"

"I'm an alcoholic. I had a relapse."

"Beyond that."

"There's nothing beyond that. If I were in remission from cancer and had a recurrence, would you ask me why I got cancer again?"

He gave me a long look, wrote something down. Shifted in his chair.

I continued. "You know as well as I do that alcoholics drink because they are alcoholics. I drink, therefore I am. We don't need a reason. That's the whole point of the disease model of addiction. Drinking *is* the problem not the symptom."

Another long look. He was making me uncomfortable.

"I noticed you say your mom has Alzheimer's."

"That's right. We've started to look for a memory care unit for her since it's not safe for her to live alone. The other day she..." I stopped myself.

"Go on."

"I know where you're going with this. I don't need a reason to drink. Maybe an excuse or a rationalization, and that could be my mom, that could be the weather, that could be the Yankees bullpen blowing another game, but it's not the reason. The reason is that I am an alcoholic. Let's leave my mom's situation out of this."

"I think that's an oversimplification. I also think you're being evasive."

"Thank you. I'll take your comments under consideration."

"And defensive."

Mentally, I stuck my tongue out at him.

"You don't have to stay here in this facility, you know. You don't even have to talk to me."

I sat back and stared at him. A moment passed.

"I'm guessing, Mr. Grinnan..."

"Edward."

"I'm guessing as the youngest, especially after the death of an older brother with challenges, you may have grown especially close to your mother, and she to you. And to see her decline like this must be very upsetting, even frightening. You're talking about a primal relationship."

"It's hard, yes. But I'm not going to drink over it. I drank when she was sharp as a pin."

"What I'm saying is that we all have triggers, things that unleash certain feelings we don't want to face, and feelings are what make us drink and get high and act out in any number of ways. A trigger is not a reason or an excuse or weakness. It's a catalyst that puts certain emotions in play that make us very uncomfortable, and for an alcoholic that can be perilous. We don't like uncomfortable emotions. Sometimes we fear our emotions. That's when we can relapse."

I nodded. I knew what he was getting at. I'd pondered it myself but resisted the notion that I started drinking because I was losing my mom to dementia. Joe wasn't drinking. Mary Lou wasn't drinking. What was my excuse?

"I'm not a therapist," Carl said, "so I don't want to go too deep into this. You might consider working with someone who is or talking to a sponsor, or a pastor, if you're into that. Personally, I don't believe you can get sober without God."

I nodded, relieved that the evaluation was apparently concluding. For the first time since I came through those red doors, I found myself thinking about a drink.

"We'll probably discharge you in a day or two with a recommendation that you continue with AA and possibly therapy. I can give you some names. I don't think you need to go back into rehab at this point. You know most of what they teach you there already. You just need to apply it. Start counting days again. This is day one."

I smiled. I liked the sound of that. The time when I first got sober in AA was one of the most wonderful periods of my life and I loved counting off the days and hearing the applause. A spiritual growth spurt. I found myself really believing, perhaps for the first time in my life, that there was a God who believed in me. Did he still?

"I have a question," I said. "I've read a few things and I wonder if you know if there is any research that says a history of alcoholism and head injury makes one more susceptible to Alzheimer's later in life?"

"Are you worried about that?"

"A little."

"Why?"

"I see it all over my family."

"It scares you even though you are still relatively young?"

"I've begun thinking about it."

"Well, I haven't seen any specific data but I wouldn't be at all surprised. Alcoholism assaults the brain and kills brain cells. The damage can be permanent. But one thing I can tell you, Edward, is this: Alcoholism makes you more susceptible to death."

I went back out to the day room. Della pointed to my lunch tray, still covered, sitting on a table. She and Tony and the guy with the Walkman were all dancing to Sly coming through the headphones.

Della waved for me to join in, but I declined and pretended to eat my lunch, tapping my foot to the bass line. "I want to thank you for lettin' me be myself..."

"Some man came by looking for you," Della said over her shoulder.

I nearly dropped my fork.

"'Cept they don't let anyone in who's not authorized. You have to have a pass."

It could only have been Fulton Oursler, my boss and the editor-in-chief of *Guideposts*. Julee must have called him. Fulton himself was an alcoholic with long-term sobriety in AA. He had been a help to me and would be even more so in the coming days and weeks. I'm glad they turned him away, though. Fulton was a force to be reckoned with. I wasn't ready to face him. I wasn't sure I was ready to face anyone. In fact, I sensed I was getting a little too comfortable with this dingy detox on the West Side of Manhattan. *How long could I hide out here?* I found myself wondering as Della pulled me out onto the impromptu dance floor.

I was let loose the next morning. Della was already gone. I guess her ship had come in via direct deposit. What a world. My hands were still a little shaky and my brain befogged. I went to a meeting before I even went home, raised my hand that still had that plastic hospital wristband on it, and sang out, "I'm Edward, I'm an alcoholic, and I have two days." I thought it would bruise my pride after having so much sober time under my belt. It didn't. It felt like a little measure of grace, a day at a time.

I wish I could say I made it to ninety—I didn't. I had to start over a couple times before I got there. On April 3, 1996, I had my last drink, God willing. I didn't know it was my last drink at the time. You never really know, do you? But by the grace of God, a day at a time, I have been sober since.

continued on p. 159

• • •

GOD HAS A way of doing things behind your back. I don't mean that irreverently. I mean that He has a way of putting you in the right place at the right time with the right person, the importance of which you are not necessarily meant to recognize or understand until much later in your life. Such was the case with a story I did with the great but troubled Glen Campbell and his wife, Kim.

I went out to Branson, Missouri, to interview Glen for *Guideposts* when I was still in the final days of my drinking, shortly before I got sober. Frankly, the circumstances made me feel a bit of an imposter since Glen had recently announced his own sobriety.

When I met Glen, he was sprawled on a couch in his rented condo, a Martin guitar at his side and a Titleist putter waggling in his hands. He had on a studio-quality set of headphones and didn't notice when Kim let me into their condo. The night before, I'd attended a concert at his temporary Branson theater. It had been an interesting show. The first half was a spirited romp through his greatest hits—"Wichita Lineman," "Galveston," "By the Time I Get to Phoenix"—played with such gusto that it was clear he still loved every note of Jimmy Webb's classic compositions. It's a wonderful thing to see a great artist who never tires of his material. It was decades after these hits had charted, decades filled with Glen's alcohol and cocaine abuse, a broken marriage, a declining career, but Glen was still the Rhinestone Cowboy glittering under the stage lights, with that Martin slung over his shoulder. He was more than a great artist. He was a great entertainer.

The second half of the show took a peculiar turn. I didn't quite know what to make of it. It was Webb's impressionistic Christian allegory based loosely on the Book of Revelation featuring modern dancers, dramatic sound, and lighting effects, and not too much Glen Campbell. It lasted about a half hour and seemed weirdly incongruous for a place like Branson, which was like Vegas without the vice, wholesome as can be but glitzy in its Ozarks way.

When Kim welcomed me into their condo, which overlooked a slightly burned-out golf course, she explained Glen was listening to a recording of the previous night's show, seeing where there might be improvements.

He noticed me and took off the headphones and shook my hand. I really wanted to ask Glen about the second act quasi-religious extravaganza. I never got the chance. We discussed his wild days and his subsequent sobriety, his immersive re-baptism in a creek near his boyhood home of Delight, Arkansas, by his pastor brother. Just as I got around to asking him about the strange second act of his show, I noticed Glen staring longingly out his picture window at the golf course and twirling his putter. He had grown increasingly distracted, pacing and practicing his putting while he talked, sometimes seeming not to hear my questions so that Kim would prompt him or answer herself.

"I think I've taken up enough of your day off, Glen," I said, putting away my notes.

He smiled and said, "Pleasure to talk with you, Edward. Kim and I are real fans of *Guideposts* and Dr. Peale." And with that he pulled his clubs from a closet and was out the door.

"He's a little ADD after six days of performing and eight shows," Kim said with a laugh. "And golf is the one addiction he'll never kick."

Kim and I talked over coffee for another hour or so. She told me how incredibly hard it was for Glen to kick cocaine and booze. "Addiction had a stranglehold on his life," she said, "until he gave himself completely to God. It was a miracle."

Branson was the start of the road back. It wasn't always a smooth road. Glen stumbled along the way, much as I did, sometimes quite publicly, but Kim was always with him, just like the music of Jimmy Webb.

Kim's Rhinestone Cowboy left us in 2017 after a long struggle with Alzheimer's. I never got to ask about that strange interpretation of Revelation that I saw in Branson or why Glen performed it. I remember it ended with a staged reenactment of a violent storm that shook the theater to its rafters, followed by a sunrise and a last number by Glen. I don't remember the song. It wasn't one of his hits. But I remember him standing alone in the center of the stage as the spotlight ever so slowly faded. There was a long silence before the audience rose to its feet and applauded. The applause lasted far longer than the silence.

I wonder now what effect Glen's addiction might have had on his eventually developing Alzheimer's. Did the booze and the coke prime his neurons for dementia? Although he would not be diagnosed with the disease for another dozen years after I interviewed him, I also wonder if his restlessness and lack of concentration that day might have been early signals of the disease rather than just the result of the rigors of his performance schedule. Had I been led to do this interview in preparation for some of my own questions and struggles that lay ahead? Could I have known at the time that Glen would become a great inspiration for me?

Kim and Glen did the world a great service by being so open about his dementia. Even as the disease progressed Glen performed for as long as he was able, even when Jimmy Webb's lyrics eluded him at times. It was both heartbreaking and inspiring to see and incredibly brave of him to get up on stage. I feel privileged to have spent some time with him, even if I was keeping him from his golf game.

IN THE YEARS SINCE, AND ESPECIALLY PREPARING FOR this book, I have poked around in the research to find out if alcohol abuse and withdrawal seizures raise your chances of developing Alzheimer's, especially in the context of a family tendency toward dementia. Certainly, there are specific dementias associated with alcoholism.

Long-term abuse of alcohol inevitably wreaks havoc on brain cells, and there is some evidence that it can indeed increase one's chances of developing Alzheimer's, though the mechanism of this connection is not completely understood. It is known that chronic heavy drinking shrinks the volume of the brain's white matter, especially within the frontal lobes, which impairs the brain's ability to perform executive functions. The symptoms produced by this damage can closely mimic the symptoms of Alzheimer's, including memory impairment.

A common alcohol-related dementia is Wernicke-Korsakoff syndrome, essentially a depletion of the B vitamin thiamine. This occurs because chronic alcoholics often eat a poor diet compounded by the fact that alcohol inhibits the absorption of B vitamins, particularly B1 or thiamine, which is why some doctors suggest taking a B vitamin supplement after a night of heavy drinking to mitigate the effects of a hangover.

Thiamine deficiency over a long period of time damages the brain. Some of that damage can be reversed if addressed early enough. There is a threshold though, where the damage is irreversible and causes a form of dementia that includes confabulation and memory impairment, motor control issues, apathy, and disorientation. Untreated, Wernicke-Korsakoff can lead to death.

One doctor I talked to advised me that I was worrying too much. "You are more than twenty-five years alcohol-free," he said. "That counts for a lot. We are resilient creatures. I've seen amazing results when alcoholics quit drinking. What's bad for your entire body, brain especially, is stress and anxiety."

And bad for the soul as well. In twelve-step programs, the spiritual goal is the attainment of serenity and spiritual well-being through a closer relationship with your Higher Power. Instead of looking at pictures of diseased brains on medical websites and wondering how mine compares, I am much better off thanking God for the blessing of sobriety and growing closer to Him in my daily spiritual practices, including prayer and meditation, and working my twelve-step program. Only God knows the future and He is waiting for me there just as He is with me today, to hold and be held.

• • •

I have mentioned the humble slogans you see posted on the walls of twelve-step meetings. They are almost simplistic in their messages. Beginners often have trouble taking them seriously (I did). And yet they have helped saved generations of alcoholics and I think they can help anyone deal with the problems of life. Here are just a few of my favorites:

- **One Day at a Time**

- **Keep it Simple (or KISS—Keep it Simple, Stupid!)**

- **Progress, Not Perfection**

- **First Things First**

- **But for the Grace of God**

- **Easy Does It**

- **Live and Let Live**

- **Let Go and Let God**

The simplicity of the slogans eventually humbled me, which was the transformation I needed. Their very simplicity focused me on turning my will and my life over to God. Left to my own devices, I would have complicated a very fundamental proposition: God loves me and wants the best for my life as long as I allow Him in unconditionally.

Every AA meeting ends with the Serenity Prayer and I will end this chapter with it. *God, grant me the serenity to accept the things I cannot change, to change the things I can and the wisdom to know the difference.*

It was a plea I would cling to in the time to come.

CHAPTER EIGHT

LOVE KNOWS NO DISTANCE

I t was around this point in my mother's decline, after my stint in detox and my conversation with the counselor, that I reluctantly agreed to see a therapist. I picked Annette from the recommendations on my counselor's list, as much an alphabetical choice as anything else. Annette was an older woman who had handled just about every kind of problem that had come through her practice, especially patients with substance use disorder, the currently preferred clinical term that seems conceived to extract the stigma from addiction and even leave a little room for an ordered return to the relevant substance. That I knew could never be true for me. I doubt many things about myself, my talents, my honesty, even my faith from time to time, but never that I am an alcoholic.

Her office was on a high floor of an older building on Central Park West whose exterior deceptively surpassed its interior. It must have once been a fairly swanky residence but now most of the spaces were taken up by medical offices, clinics, foundations, and lots of shrinks. The elevator was slow and clanky and made me wish I had taken the steps, which would have gotten my heart rate up but my anxiety level down. But Annette's office was comfortable if well-used, nicely appointed, with two walls of bookcases groaning under the weight of their contents. Always a good sign. Annette was warm and welcoming but not enough to put much of a dent in my wariness. It had been quite a few years since I'd seen a therapist, and I'd never done so voluntarily. Part of me thought seeing a shrink would only make matters worse, deconstructing the defenses I'd carefully erected for basic survival.

I was resistant at first, as most patients are to therapy, even those who throw themselves into it quite willingly but don't really know what they're in for. I went because a number of people in my life had insisted on it, and I was in no position to refuse. Besides, I was growing increasingly anxious about being so far away from my mother when she needed so much. I knew I needed to deal with that anxiety.

Therapy is primarily a process of gaining self-knowledge. I went into it thinking I knew everything about myself that I cared to know (Freud once said that the Irish were the only people who were completely impervious to psychoanalysis). Yet as I talked, week after week, I realized what I mostly knew was biography. Stories. When it came to examining the feelings behind that biography and those stories, I was insanely resistant. "It is what it is. Feelings don't matter that much. They're just reactions."

"That's what you think," Annette would say. Usually, she smiled when she said it.

"This isn't helping me," I complained to my AA sponsor. "I'm just blabbering about myself."

"You don't know that," he said. "The closer you get to some truth about yourself, the more you want to quit. Every time. Remember, AA is a program of suggestions and I strongly suggest you stick with it." I knew he might drop me if I didn't, suggestion or no suggestion.

So, I did, schlepping twice weekly up to Annette's building with the deceptive exterior and deteriorating interior. And yes, friends, it did occur to me that that might be a metaphor.

"I'm neglecting my work for these sessions," I protested to her one day.

"Your work. That's interesting. Tell me more about that."

"Mostly I help other people tell their stories for the magazine."

"How do you do that?" Annette asked.

"Well, you want the basics of the story, of course, the structure of the narrative. Storytelling at its most basic is simply the structure of information. The storyteller is like a card dealer. Each card they turn over is another piece of information that advances the narrative, which keeps the reader reading. The real work comes from digging deeper, digging deeper into the narrator's emotions, how they felt about the experience they're sharing with our readers, how they've been changed by it spiritually, what they learned about themselves and their faith. It's about gaining insight. You're as much a therapist as an editor." I wanted to take that last statement back, but it was too late. She smiled.

"So, the emotions are the key that unlocks the story."

"You could say that."

I knew I was painting myself into a corner; we weren't yet halfway through the session. I don't normally sweat from nervousness, but I could feel my brow getting damp. I was shifting around in my chair more than usual. Writhing, you could say.

"Do you write this way about yourself ever?"

"Not really. Usually, I write for others who need help telling their stories." I paused. "Lately I've been trying my hand at devotions for our annual devotional book. Devotions are little true stories with a spiritual lesson embedded in them. My editor is pressuring me to write something from my point of view."

"Pressuring you?"

"I thought it would be an interesting challenge. A writing challenge. To branch out…nothing I'd want to do on an ongoing basis."

"I see. So do your emotions unlock the story?"

"I suppose they do, as a writing technique, at least."

We paused. I hated these pauses. My tendency is to fill the air with words.

"You know what I'm getting at," she said. "It's obvious."

"Perhaps." I folded my arms. Yes, maybe Freud was on to something. There was an interval of silence, like the silence between movements of a symphony.

Annette broke the spell. "Maybe the way to reach your emotions is through writing, writing about yourself, honestly, though I imagine that's the hard part, especially for you, who finds your emotions in the stories of others. Tell me about one of your devotions."

I stared out the big, leaded window that looked out over Central Park West through a grimy film, the faint sound of horns as taxis jockeyed for position like swarming yellow beetles, a perfect example of chaos theory in action.

"Okay. I wrote one about my mother losing her memory and how hard it was to see that, especially from a distance, as if there was nothing I could do. It was about feeling powerless."

"Angry?"

"Devotions aren't really about anger."

Annette gave me a skeptical look. "But powerlessness is. Could you do anything about your mother's dementia if you were there?"

"Probably not. Maybe it would make me feel better."

"So instead, you stay here where you have a support system, have a job that helps people and helps you, a wife and two dogs you love. Do you think your mother would want that life for you?"

I nodded.

"How did the story end?"

"My devotion? Well, with prayer, I guess. The devotion ends with a prayer asking God to help me with this burden of my conscience and to comfort my mom." Then I added, feeling myself backtrack, "The prayer is a convention of the form."

Oh no, I thought, *she's giving me that smile again.*

Annette never talked much about faith, and I could only guess what hers was if any. She was a shrink, not a pastor, and somehow she made that clear without proclaiming it. Today was different, if only because she might have found a way in.

"You believe in prayer," she said, as a statement.

"I try very hard to."

"You pray for what when it comes to this situation with your mother?"

"I don't know. That she does not suffer. That I be given the wisdom to know how to handle the situation. That I stay sober."

"Are you afraid?"

"Yes. For my mom." I stopped. "For myself too, I guess. I'm so much like her."

"You're afraid this will happen to you someday?"

"It's so selfish...and I've already done so much damage already. I have only myself to blame."

"Why blame anyone?"

I didn't have an answer, at least not one I was willing to share.

"Prayer," she said, "is not really about the prayer, whatever you're praying for. It's about trust, trust in your faith, trust you are being heard, trust that you are not alone. Prayer is about trust more than answers. Sometimes it is the only healthy way to channel your anger, at a power so much larger than your anger. Edward, I think you are angry because you are afraid. Anger is fear turned inside out."

Annette was coming perilously close to giving me advice, which she never did. She wanted me to find my own answers, like any good therapist.

"You are on a journey of trust," she said after a moment. "Trust in your prayers, trust in your family, trust in your sobriety, trust in yourself, which you must find. Most of all, trust in love. You love your mother, you love your family, and they love you, you love yourself, presumably. That love will protect you as well as help you. Love is the strongest thing there is. It gives life meaning. Without it we die. Maybe you'll discover it in your writing, writing for yourself instead of ventriloquizing other people."

That last bit stung, but in a good way. For a minute I thought I would cry. That would be a first in this room. In the beginning I used to accuse Annette of just trying to get me to cry with her questions. Yet wasn't that what I did with a good *Guideposts* story? To bring a tear to the reader's eye? Julee would sometimes tease me about having a job that made people cry. Yes, I'd say, but it's good crying. Catharsis. Emotional release. Empathy. And besides, her music made some people cry. I wasn't the only guilty one.

"I'll leave you with one last thing to think about, Edward. Love knows no distance."

• • •

ITHOUGHT A LOT ABOUT THE FACT THAT love knows no distance. But that didn't make it any easier to be far away. I would hear stories about what Mom was doing, and I would try to accept that I couldn't always be there.

There are moments that I think back on now that make me smile, even laugh, though they probably shouldn't. Still, most families have these kinds of stories.

One June Saturday, for instance, my mother was in her yard gardening, at the house next to Joe and Toni's. Gardening was something she loved to do not just for the horticultural rewards but for the hard dirty work it occasioned. Mom was a ball of energy and she liked to stay physically busy: gardening, shoveling snow, mowing the lawn, jogging, scrubbing the kitchen floor. When she relaxed—or put her feet up, as she liked to say—it was usually with a book or the newspaper.

On this particular Saturday, in the midst of her gardening, she was evidently seized by the notion that she needed to go to church. Immediately. Having lost her driver's license, she set out for St. Owen's, several miles away, on foot. Remember, she was 80 years old by now and it was a warm day.

According to witness accounts, she more or less barged into the church, marched up the main aisle, and made her way to the altar. It's hard to know what she was thinking. Maybe she felt the altar flowers needed tending, or the altar cloths changing. She was still in her gardening clothes and had her trowel in her hand, mind you.

The problem was there was a wedding ceremony being conducted and the bride and groom were exchanging vows when my mother appeared and started wandering around the altar, her face sweaty and dirt-smeared.

Fortunately, her friend and protector, Sister Carolyn, was on hand and was able to quickly rectify the situation and the wedding continued, though not without more than a few mouths agape. Sister called Joe, who came and got Mom. It was difficult to elicit an explanation from Mom for her behavior. Our working theory is that she suddenly thought she was late for 5 p.m. Saturday Mass and panicked, rushing to church before it was too late.

There is nothing funny about Alzheimer's. Yet there are things you can't help but laugh about, if only to preserve your sanity. When Mary Lou called me about this episode, I caught myself smiling at the image of my mother, trowel in hand, invading the wedding. My mother was so headstrong she was going to attend Mass no matter what anyone else had planned, damn it. Besides, it would give the bride and groom something to talk about for years to come. "Remember when that lady crashed our wedding...."

• • •

LIKE MANY PEOPLE WITH ALZHEIMER'S, MY MOTHER EXPERIENCED a lowering of inhibitions and filters, not that my mother wasn't outspoken to begin with. Mary Lou remembers taking her to Easter brunch after church where she loudly demanded to be fed immediately. "I'm hungry. I have to eat. I have to eat right now!" My mom was never the most patient person, but she was never rude or inconsiderate. Quite the opposite, really. Since both Mary Lou and I had waited tables during our college days, and me much later, she was unfailingly considerate to servers.

The one moment that still makes me laugh every time I think of it is when I was visiting her at Clausen one trip back to Michigan. She got along with the staff very well, except for one lady. I was in Mom's room with her when this particular aide brought Mom a fresh carafe of ice water, which she had been urged to drink due to her borderline dehydration.

"There you go, Estelle," the aide said pleasant as could be and turned to leave.

"Thanks a lot," Mom said, "...fat ass."

I had never heard my mother swear or even say that word. I could barely hold it together and when I returned to my rental car in the parking lot later, I laughed until I cried. I'm sure people must have thought I was shedding tears of anguish instead of laughing hysterically at a side of my mother I never knew existed. In fact, does Alzheimer's change us or does it just peel back the layers of our identity?

• • •

NOT LONG AFTER THE WEDDING INCIDENT AT ST. Owen's there was a far more disturbing and mystifying occurrence. One morning Toni and Joe sent Clare and Rachel over to Mom's with some baked goods. They returned just a few minutes later.

"There was a fire at Grandma's house," Clare said.

Toni and Joe rushed over. Mom seemed calm, almost oblivious. She didn't have much of an explanation to share.

And the fire certainly needed an explanation because it was not a small event. It was a miracle the house hadn't burned to the ground. Apparently, the fire started in a staircase that led to an attic space that Mom often haunted, looking for what no one ever knew, least of all her. She would rummage through things, a behavioral manifestation of what must have been going through her mind, searching for the parts of herself that were disappearing, as if she was trying to find out who she was, an echo of King Lear: "Who is it that can tell me who I am?"

The walls and ceiling were scorched and charred, and the smell of smoke still hung in the air. There was evidence Mom might have tried to throw some water on the blaze but clearly it would have taken more than that to put it out. Much more. This had been a real fire.

How it started was as much a mystery as how it was extinguished. Mom didn't use candles or anything like that. My father had forbidden it, given his own fire phobia. Maybe a lamp fell over, Mom didn't notice or forgot about it, and the hot bulb set fire to some of the piles of papers she was muddling through. There were half-emptied boxes everywhere, giving Mom a good excuse to complain about having to move in the first place and try to find something.

"There was nothing wrong with my other house. I could find anything." She paced back and forth in the living room talking to herself, as Joe and Toni inspected the damage.

How had the house not burned down? A fire doesn't put itself out.

"Mom, did you call the fire department?" Joe asked, though it was difficult to believe a fire crew could have come out in the middle of the night without Joe and Toni noticing.

"Two men in a car stopped. They helped me."

"Two men?"

"Yes, they put the fire out."

"Then what?"

"Then they left."

"Did they say who they were?"

"No."

"Did you ask?"

"I don't remember."

"Were they firemen?"

"No, I don't think so. They wore suits and ties."

"Police?"

"I don't think so."

"Just two men?"

"Yes."

"And they just...left?"

"I think so."

Mom's house was far enough back from the road that it was unlikely anyone would have noticed flames coming from the inside. As much as Joe and Toni probed, they couldn't get anything more than the story about the two mysterious men. There was no use pushing her. She was growing more anxious and defensive. At some level Mom knew something dangerous had happened, maybe the result of something she shouldn't have been doing, especially in the middle of the night.

I think Mom sensed she should have been able to explain the incident and was upset she couldn't, that it was all so confusing. This is one of the worst things about the mid stages of dementia, experts say. The sufferer knows her mind is slipping and is trying desperately to hold on, to grasp for some explanation. Yet confusion begets confusion. Anxiety fuels greater anxiety.

Beverly Hills, Michigan, is a fairly small community and Joe and Toni were pretty well connected. They checked with the fire chief and the fire department. They hadn't responded to a fire at my mother's address. They checked with the cops. No record of a fire with them either. They talked to neighbors. No one saw a car with two men stop. No one saw anything. Yet my mom insisted, when questioned again, that two men appeared to put out the fire. Then she went to bed after they left.

"Are you sure a couple of kids out late didn't stop?" I asked Joe when he called.

"It doesn't seem plausible," he said.

I wracked my mind for an explanation but couldn't come up with anything except that Mom's situation was getting increasingly dangerous.

We never solved the mystery. Mary Lou was sure she knew, though. "I think they were angels," she said. "Angels that came to protect Mom. It's the only explanation."

• • •

AFTER MY SESSION WITH ANNETTE I CROSSED OVER Central Park West and entered the park, walking aimlessly as the sun set, the fading light feeling good on my back as shadows lengthened, cutting across the thick green grass and the walkways.

I passed the Naumburg Bandshell and found myself stopping at the Bethesda Fountain, staring up at the Angel of the Water surrounded by her cherubic handmaidens, Temperance, Purity, Health, and Peace (not to be confused with Patience and Fortitude, the guardian lions of the New York Public Library on Fifth Avenue).

The eight-foot bronze figure towers above cascading waters, reaching down to touch them, an homage to the healing waters of the Biblical pool described in John 5:2–4 (NKJV). "Now there is in Jerusalem by the Sheep *Gate* a pool, which is called in Hebrew, Bethesda, having five porches. In these lay a great multitude of sick people...waiting for the moving of the water. For an angel went down at a certain time into the pool and stirred up the water; then whoever stepped in...was made well..."

There was to be no miracle for my mother, for no one has ever survived Alzheimer's, and I understood but could not quite allow myself to accept that she was not going to be the first. Was a miracle just a matter of luck? Or did faith itself bring healing? Could love of God help free one from suffering or grant one the grace to bear it? A deliverance rather than an old-fashioned Biblical healing. Is love the one miracle we always have?

The water was New York City drinking water. At the bottom of the pool was a scattering of coins for good luck. The fountain is possibly the most beautiful structure in Central Park, a monument to the perseverance of hope and prayer, rendered from everyday things.

I dipped my hand into the water, held it in front of me, and let the water run through my fingers, a shaft of fading sunlight hitting it just so, almost like a tiny rainbow. It takes about eight minutes for the light of the sun, its congregation of photons, to reach the earth traveling at 300,000 kilometers a second. We say that things happen at the speed of light, which is to say virtually instantly. Except light travels a great distance at the exact same speed, say from a galaxy five billion light-years away, meaning it takes the light five billion years to reach us, virtually the age of our planet. It's easy then to think of light travelling not instantaneously but majestically, a slow rolling wave of pure matterless energy plying the cosmos.

Can love too travel distance similarly? The love of two people joined, the love of people at a distance, the love from heaven, the love from God. Does the velocity of love cover all distance in different ways?

Walking home I thought more about what Annette said about love knowing no distance. Clearly, she meant I loved my mother as much from afar as near. Yet something else suddenly struck me. As Alzheimer's extracts its toll on the sufferer, you care for them from a distance even if you are right at their bedside. They drift further away from us as the disease progresses. We are there but they are not. Inevitably we care for them at a distance no matter where we are.

Yet we yearn to be present, which is not always possible in a country as large as the U.S. with a population as dispersed as we are. People live farther from their hometowns than ever before. And let's face it, travel can be a real hassle these days, right?

continued on p. 180

• • •

A FEW YEARS ago, the newsman Richard Lui sat for an interview with *Guideposts* for one of the magazine's special sections on Alzheimer's caregiving. He grew up in San Francisco, where his father was a pastor, social worker, and beloved member of the community. In recent years, his father has suffered cognitive decline and memory loss.

Richard, who is based in New York, has juggled his career at NBC with caring for his dad and also acting as a spokesperson for the Alzheimer's Association. That's a lot of balls to keep in the air and I was honored that he was so generous with his time. In the interview that follows, reprinted from the April 2019 issue of *Guideposts*, Richard shares his experience as a long-distance caregiver and offers some of the very best advice I have heard on the topic.

Your dad, Stephen, was a pastor, social worker, and vibrant part of his community. When did you notice that something wasn't right with him?

Dad was a prayer guy. At our big family Christmas gathering, he always said this elaborate prayer that would take him a week to prepare. At the end he'd say, "Turn to your relatives to the left and the right and hug them and tell them why you love them." Seven years ago, when he gave his prayer, he forgot his siblings' names. For decades, he had done this prayer. It was a big deal for the entire Lui clan that he couldn't do it. My aunt took me aside and said, "I think your dad should see a doctor." He'd always been very open to understanding sickness. And I think something about him was like, "I'm sick. Let me go and try to fix this." He went in and got diagnosed, and he never was down about it.

You, along with your three siblings and your mom, are part of your dad's caregiving team. They all live in California, and you fly in from New York. Besides visiting every few weeks, what are some of the ways you keep in contact?

We created a Google doc and list all of his doctors' appointments, test results, medicines, activities, visitors, etc. It's really helpful to have everything in one place so we don't have to constantly call to ask for updates.

Anything else?

If you're not sure where your loved one is in the disease, stay overnight. Don't go for a meal or special occasion. Stay overnight because the bumps in the night are often more than bumps in the night. You won't know the cause if you're not there. I'd always stay overnight in the room I grew up in. And the days I wasn't there, my mom told me my dad would go by my room, open the door, and say, "Good night, Richard. Good night."

What advice do you have for long-distance caregivers who get distressed if they can't visit their loved ones?

Just own that it's hard. Accept that you're not perfect. Talk to someone about it. I think the biggest stress is, *Am I making the right decision? If I stick with my job or don't? If I call in sick? If I don't see my family or my friends or my significant other? What is the right thing?* And I think the struggle is thinking, *I will never make the right decision. I'm in a no-win situation.* But actually, you are in an always-win decision if you are keeping your loved one in mind and what they would want you to do. Check out the Alzheimer's Association website, alz.org, as well for great info and resources for caregivers.

You've found that caregiving doesn't have to be serious all the time. How has humor helped you and your family?

Finding some humor in all of this is very human and very necessary and doesn't take away the difficulty, the sadness. When he was diagnosed, Dad was active and able to take care of himself. Now, seven years later, he's living in a care facility. He's bedridden and can't feed himself. We are dealing with tough stuff. When he was still living at home and I started having to change him and clean him, he loved to run around the house naked. Sometimes he'd go, "Oh, I have to poop." Boy, cleaning up his poop and helping with diapers—that freaked me out. I knew this was a benchmark when Dad couldn't take care of himself. I started to joke about it. And I hope it helped my siblings. We would use the poop emoji in our group texts when we took turns watching him. "Oh, he pooped today." Then we would use one, two, three, or four poop emojis. "He did a three. He did a two. He did a one." It was really tough for my one brother who's super clean and doesn't like to talk about that stuff. But even he started to joke along with us.

You had to start shaving your father as well. That must have been difficult.

Dad had a morning ritual. Get up, eat his oats and milk and raisins. And shave. There came a point where he didn't know how to do it anymore. I took out his electric razor. When I turned it on, he smiled. He liked the feel of it on his skin. And he squealed—*whoo* and *yeah*—like a kid. Dad had taught me how to shave, and I thought it was very symbolic of that shift of roles we go through, helping parents with Alzheimer's. It was not only that I was shaving him but that it meant so much to him. I held his hand throughout the entire process. It was a moment of connection.

How has your faith helped you as caregiver?

It's definitely been a source of strength and comfort for me. We're pastor's kids. My eldest sibling texted in our group thread that he had just read John, chapter one, to Dad. We're each reading a chapter when we visit. We pick up where the last sibling or Mom left off. For Dad, sound is definitely key. He loves the Lord and the Bible, and he can also hear and recognize our voices.

He can't talk anymore, but he does interact. When he's keyed in, his eyes will look at you. He'll smile.

Can you talk more about the importance of voice, sounds, and music for your dad?

We can speak into an amplifier or have it play sounds. The connected headphones act as hearing aids. My dad was always hard of hearing. With Alzheimer's, his senses need all the help they can get.

You've said that watching the progression of Alzheimer's was like watching your dad die a bit in front of you. And then being born again. Can you explain?

Dad was a real stressed-out guy when he was middle-aged. He took home all the problems of people he was trying to help as a social worker and a pastor. I think he was born again in that, despite this disease being part of his new life, he hasn't gone back to worrying. He's so positive. He's the most wonderful patient. All the nurses love him because he would kiss everybody on the hand and smile and laugh with them. Life is a stack of pancakes, and Alzheimer's takes the top pancakes little by little until you're left with none. Even if this disease has stripped away all his memories like pancakes, well, look at him. Dad is a good, faithful man.

Editor's note: This story was published in our April 2019 issue. Richard's father passed away at the age of 88 in December 2021.

MY DAD WAS A GOOD, FAITHFUL MAN, IF stern and distant. Except when it came to my brother Bobby, who was the apple of his eye and upon whom he doted. When Bobby was born, the nuns offered to take him away to a place where "children like him" could be cared for. My mom said it was the only time she thought my father would ever slug a nun. God gave Bobby to our family for a reason. When Bobby turned up dead it broke my father's heart. Literally. He had cardiac problems for the rest of his life. And as hard as it is to believe I don't think he ever blamed or was angry at God. He saw those twelve years of Bobby's life as a gift. And however much he and I came into conflict later in life, I never forgot the depth of his love for Bobby.

He loved Bobby more than he loved me because Bobby needed that love more. I was the accidental late-in-life baby who was preceded by a Down syndrome baby and at least one miscarriage. Upon hearing of the pregnancy—my mother was in her forties—the priests quietly said it would be all right with the church if she had what was then called a D and C. She felt the same way about that as my father did about the meddlesome nuns. Mom needed one more little boy to love.

There was a close family friend named Gretchen who was married to one of my father's boyhood pals, John. They happened to end up near us in Michigan. John had done very, very well at GM but died before Gretchen, though she was considerably older. Eventually Gretchen developed Alzheimer's. They had no children and the nieces and nephews seemed not to care much about Gretchen except with respect to the provisions of her substantial will, of which they were the beneficiaries.

So, it was Dad, never very fond of Gretchen to be truthful, who stopped by the high-end care facility she landed in, complete with a private room and a private nurse, to visit with her every week out of an obligation to John. I'm sure he didn't relish the chore, but he knew she didn't have anyone else except us. My mom would go too when she had a chance and Joe and Toni and Mary Lou and even me on rare occasion. Gretchen could be abusive, but no one ever took it personally, though it irked my mom. Even after Gretchen forgot who my father was, he made his visits. As I said, he was a good and faithful man.

• • •

IT WAS JUST TURNING DARK WHEN I GOT home from Central Park. I wasn't sure if my mother was still awake but gave her a call anyway. "I was just finishing up the dinner dishes," she said, though I knew if she'd eaten at all it was hours ago. "I'm going to watch something on TV."

"What show?"

"Oh, I'm not sure. I'll find something. Maybe the news or something. Or Lawrence Welk. Are you going to stop by?"

"Mom, I'm in New York. I don't think Lawrence Welk is on anymore."

"Yes, I always forget." She laughed at her mistake, not in embarrassment but just at how silly it was. It was a laugh that lifted my heart.

"Love you, Mom."

"Love you too."

I hung up the phone and said a prayer of thanks. That laugh. It made me feel very close to her.

CHAPTER NINE

WHERE DO MEMORIES GO?

Where do memories go when we lose them? Do they simply disaggregate as our neurons decay? Where does the identity of that actor go—the one I see on television and whom I have seen a hundred times in movies but suddenly can't place his all-too-familiar name? I google a clue and, ah, yes! That's him! But is that a newly formed memory of his identity or the resuscitation of one that was caught in my brain all along and just needed a little excavating? We know so little, really, about how memory works.

There was an account recently concerning an eighty-seven-year-old epilepsy patient who died of cardiac arrest while undergoing an EEG (there was no connection between the electroencephalography test and the man's heart attack). An EEG records the brain's electrical activity. This was the first instance of those measurements being made at the moment of death. Doctors inadvertently got to see what happens inside a person's brain when they die. The findings were surprising. Specifically, doctors observed sudden and dramatic changes in a particular band of brain waves called gamma oscillations, known to be involved in memory retrieval. It would seem then that at the instant of death a deluge of memories is released. Our memories are the last sigh of human life. We leave this world on a tide of memory. Yet do people who have lost their memories experience this? Science cannot answer that question. Yet.

• • •

I WONDER SOMETIMES, FANCIFULLY, I CONFESS, IF THERE is some vast dimension that is the lost and found of memories. Row after eternal row of all the memories people have lost. I indulge this fantasy because memories seem too powerful, too fundamental to who we are, the neuronal gravity that holds us together and makes us human, to just disappear into some void. We often speak of sharing a memory but no two memories from two different people are exactly alike. Our memories are unique to our individual perceptions. They are ours and ours alone. How can they simply disintegrate? Memories, I believe, are a form of matter and not simply abstractions; they exist in chemical form in our brains. If we are to believe physics, matter itself is indestructible. Can memories be destroyed? Maybe that is why I want to believe there is some great cosmic lost and found where all memories survive even when we have forgotten them, perhaps to be restored to us by God.

As Alzheimer's destroys a person's capacity to remember, to store and use information, the capacity to think is undermined to the point that for all practical purposes, the conscious mind ceases to function. We literally forget how to think. It is at this point that families must consider relinquishing their suffering loved one to the care of professionals better able to provide the intensive care that is now needed. For my family that decision seemed obvious, in retrospect at least. At the time it wasn't. It was hard. It's always hard.

continued on p. 187

• • •

IWROTE A number of devotions for our annual devotional *Walking in Grace* about my mother's plight and the decisions my family faced. I like to think that a writer named Donna Teti might have read some of them.

A few years later she wrote a moving and surprisingly uplifting story about her own family's decision to put their mother, Jean, in a care facility. I like the story not just for its reassuring quality but for the fact that it takes place in a very brief period of time with a resounding spiritual lesson. Sometimes the more compact the story the bigger the takeaway.

That day Donna pulled a chair up to the table where her mom was eating lunch with some other residents and asked in a voice more cheerful than she felt, "How's lunch, Mom?"

Donna had chosen to climb the three flights of stairs to her mother's floor instead of taking the elevator in the hopes the knot in her stomach would ease. Even after all these months and despite the fact that her mother had both dementia and cancer and needed advanced care, more care than Donna and her siblings could possibly provide at home, she still felt tormented by the decision to place her here, a decision they prayed hard about. To a daughter who loved her mother, it still held the echo of betrayal.

The dining room smelled like a grade-school cafeteria. "Delicious!" her mother finally said. *At least her attitude is good today,* Donna thought. *Be grateful for that.*

Donna updated her mom on the doings of her grand-children, repeating information as quickly as her mother forgot it. The other ladies chimed in with information about their children and grandchildren, which Donna pretended to be hearing for the first time. She smiled, nodded.

Her mother's gaze scanned the room until it landed on a favorite aide, Janelle. "I love her," she said. "She is soooo beautiful." Janelle waved and for an instant Donna could glimpse the mother she remembered...kind, gra-cious, generous. Then her mom's smile turned to a scowl. "I need more milk," she demanded petulantly.

"You already had your milk, Mom," Donna said, holding up the empty carton.

"Here," Elsa, Donna's mother's roommate said, "she can have mine," and slid her carton over with a straw. "She won't drink it without a straw." Donna smiled. Her mother was a lifelong straw drinker.

Lunch concluded, Donna wheeled her mother into the lobby area where others were. Her mother was im-patient now. "I want to go to sleep."

Donna couldn't get her mom into bed on her own and all the aides were occupied with other residents. She felt so helpless! Her mom wanted to rest, and all Donna could do was stand there. "I want to go to sleep," she repeated. Donna thought of all the child-hood years her mother put her to bed with a lullaby or a story. Now it had come to this.

Then over hobbled Frankie, a former mummer from south Philly and a real kidder.

"Hey, Jean," Frankie whispered, "where you going all dressed up like that?"

"I'm dressed for the cemetery," Donna's mom muttered.

"Not yet," Frankie said. "You have to stay with us in Suffering Springs!" Then he laughed.

A feeble joke, I suppose, but it got a smile out of Donna's mom and then a laugh.

"I guess so!" she said.

As Frankie launched into another joke, one he had told a hundred times before, Donna's mom leaned in. Donna knew that this was a scene that repeated itself over and over again in this place. Yet now, instead of depressing her, she felt relief. No one here had long to live but living they were. There were still jokes and laughter and smiles. Yes, Suffering Springs had its moments. Donna waved Janelle over.

"I have to go now, Mom," she said.

"Don't," her mom pleaded, and Donna pushed down the guilt as Frankie launched into another story that probably had no ending and slipped away.

Donna held back tears until she reached the car. It was so hard to see her mother like this, in a strange place with strange people. Yet, there was Frankie the jokester, an aide named Janelle her mother loved, a roommate who knew she only drank milk with a straw. They were almost like family, a new family at a time in her life when her own children could no longer care for her in that way.

Drying her tears, Donna knew that the decision to put her mom into care was the right one, one that had been guided by the prayers they said, but which made it no easier. Because these life decisions are never easy when love is involved. Love can make you do the right thing and still feel bad about it. As she drove away, no matter what her heart said, Donna knew her mom was in a good place.

T HE FINAL PART OF MY FAMILY'S JOURNEY BEGAN with a phone call my mother made one evening to 911. "There's a little boy missing. He's twelve. You have to find him."

The police were there in minutes. My mother met them in the yard and explained that she had looked everywhere, and she couldn't find her twelve-year-old son. She was frantic, pacing and wringing her hands and asking where he could have gone.

It took no time at all, of course, for the police to understand that an eighty-year-old woman could not have a twelve-year-old son. Was it her grandson? A neighbor? Was she simply confused or worse? They brought her inside the house because it was a cold spring night and tried to get the story and a phone number of someone they could call. Meanwhile they had no choice but to initiate a search plan and apprise the proper agency to prepare.

My older brother Bobby, who had Down syndrome, had disappeared on Friday the twenty-second of March 1963, just a couple years after we moved from Philadelphia to Birmingham, Michigan, a burgeoning northern suburb of Detroit. He was twelve. I can still remember being pulled from fourth-grade class at Meadow Lake School by

Mr. Shaeffer. A neighbor, Mrs. Arnold, was waiting for me in her car to take me home. I still remember all the police cars parked at our house and the local news vans that would soon arrive and the reporters I recognized from TV.

Mary Lou was there, too, in her maroon Marian High School uniform. And my father, everyone looking grim. Joe was back east in military college. I don't remember who told me Bobby was "missing" but I remember wondering exactly what that word meant in relation to my brother. Missing? How? In the house? I knew all his hiding places. I could find him in a minute.

Bobby had seemingly walked off the face of the earth. He'd gone for his usual morning ramble up Pebbleshire before the bus picked him up for his afternoon session at St. Barbara's, a special ed school. He'd chatted with some workmen building a house down the road who'd paused to eat an early lunch. Bobby had reportedly cadged half a sandwich off one of them. Then he simply wandered away. Normally he knew enough to come home in time for the bus. He was good about that. He loved the bus and going to school. But that day he never came back. When an hour had passed, my mom called my dad and then the police.

He was missing for nearly a month. Initially the police had found a puzzling set of footprints in the snow near a pump house across from the man-made lake at the center of our subdivision. They didn't lead anywhere and seemed to indicate confusion. It was difficult to tell how many sets of footprints were present as the weather was turning bad.

The next day they dusted the house for fingerprints and took ours. I can't remember if it was the FBI or local law enforcement. I'll never forget the ink on my fingers and the powder everywhere. They also searched the surface of the fake lake, which was more than a foot thick with ice and covered with undisturbed snow. The day after that they crisscrossed the lake on horseback. Later, as spring moved in, they broke through the melting ice and sent in divers. The chief of detectives, Chief Denke, who was in charge of the investigation and who had never had a minute when he wasn't thinking about it, said, "If there's one thing we're sure of, Bobby is not in that lake."

As is typical in such cases, many clues and theories surfaced. A reclusive neighbor said she saw a suspicious brown car cruising the neighborhood in the days preceding Bobby's disappearance and spotted Bobby talking to the driver once, a man with a bushy red mustache. My parents went on TV to plead for him to come home or be returned. Annette Funicello, Bobby's favorite Mouseketeer, made a similar appeal. Nobody said the word "kidnapping," but it was on everyone's mind; otherwise, it was thought, they would have found him by now. No one believed he ran away.

Clues and reports came in from all over the state and country. Our church, St. Owen's, prayed for Bobby every Sunday and our pastor, Father Walling, came by the house nearly every day to sit with my parents. There was a small item in *Time* or *Newsweek* about the case. My father followed men in brown cars who had mustaches until Chief Denke told him to stop. There was talk of bringing in the famous Dutch psychic Peter Hurkos, who had worked the Boston Strangler case. But it was too late.

I was in a movie theater watching Fred MacMurray in *Son of Flubber* when a member of our parish came and got me and took me home. Everyone was there. They'd found Bobby.

His body was floating in that lake in the center of our subdivision. Two girls walking along the shore had spotted it. Nobody could explain how he ended up there, least of all Chief Denke and his team.

Controversy ensued. The DA wanted to simply close the case. Denke wanted to keep the investigation going. The DA, an elected politician, won. He didn't want an open child disappearance and death case on the books. Chief Denke resigned in protest but stayed in touch with my parents for years, never satisfied with how the case was closed. Neither was my father.

One question always haunted my parents. When Bobby's body was found his boots were on the wrong feet, as if someone might have dressed him. Could that have been my mother? She couldn't remember, but Bobby was perfectly capable of dressing himself and putting his boots on properly. The police asked if my mother could have put the boots on and in her haste put them on the wrong feet? She just couldn't remember, but Bobby was very particular about such things and would probably have protested it, and the footprints found at the pump house did not appear to be from boots that were on the wrong feet, though it was hard to tell in the drifting snow.

My parents gave the young girl who first spotted Bobby's body floating in the lake a necklace with a small gold cross on it.

• • •

THE POLICE THAT RESPONDED TO MY MOTHER'S CALL some thirty years later had no way of knowing any of this. Had there been a reliable internet at the time—this was the early '90s—a quick data-base search would have revealed that there are several sites still focused on my brother's disappearance along with other children who subse-quently went missing and turned up dead in the years that followed. The man suspected in some of these subsequent abductions killed himself before he could be questioned.

Eventually the police got ahold of Joe and called off the search. I heard about it all the next day in a call that was hard to listen to. I remember Toni saying, "How awful for your mom's mind to be stuck in the worst memory of her life." As if it could be that singular terri-fying memory—that moment you realize your child is missing—that could survive anything, so deep and life-altering as it was that not even Alzheimer's could erase it. It was time, we all agreed, to do something.

Mary Lou said that recently Mom had been seeing things. "She told me she saw a little girl running through the house one day. I asked her if it was Clare or Rachel. She said, no, the girl was American." (My nieces Clare and Rachel were adopted from Korea and I hasten to mention they are as American as any of us.) Mom claimed the little girl then ran upstairs but there was no upstairs to that house.

"She told me how Cass was so mean to her growing up," Mary Lou said. Cass was the oldest of Mom's sisters and the first to get Alzheimer's. Mom had never spoken ill of Cass before. "She was always picking on me," Mom complained now. "She still is."

• • •

I WAS ALWAYS A LITTLE WARY MYSELF OF my aunt Cass Gallagher. There was something fierce about her, not that she was anything but kind and loving to me. She had kept a kneeler on the landing of a dark wooden staircase that led to the upper floor of her house out in Paoli at the end of the Main Line, just in case one had the urge to pray on the way up or down. Above it hung a painting of a very grim saint whose identity thankfully escapes me now and spooked me when I was young. She was an Irish partisan and hated the Beatles because they were English, and the expression "British invasion" appalled her. Plus, she thought their music sounded "exactly like the screams of the damned in hell." Her words.

Mom's other sister, Marion—also a Gallagher because she and Cass married brothers—and Cass eventually ended up in nursing homes when their dementia worsened to the point that it would have been irresponsible and inhumane to keep them at home or with family.

We were determined to find the right facility for Mom. When Cass reached the end stages of her illness she refused all food, not unexpected at that point of the disease. She was ready to die and had stopped speaking almost altogether. The one remaining option was a feeding tube, which would likely only prolong the process and came with risks. Still, the medical staff was duty bound to offer the procedure, if reluctantly.

Her family agonized over the decision until their pastor intervened and convinced them after much painful discussion that their faith required them to do all they possibly could to preserve life. So, the decision was made to use the feeding tube. As they wheeled Cass into the procedure room, she suddenly spoke the first coherent words she had spoken in months, clearly and unmistakably: "My husband never would have allowed this." They were also the last words she would ever speak. She died a short time later from an infection caused by the insertion of the feeding tube. My cousin and his family were devastated.

If there was one thing we all agreed on—me, Joe, Mary Lou, Toni, and Julee—it was that we would never resort to those extreme methods or place Mom in a facility that would use them.

• • •

THE FACILITY WE FOUND WAS TRULY A GODSEND. I use "we" loosely because it was through the determined efforts of my sister and my sister-in-law that a spot in a nearly perfect place opened up (I felt like a bystander back in New York). Toni and Mary Lou made an effective team in evaluating the numerous facilities they visited, some of which were truly horrors. When they found Lourdes Senior Community Center, they knew they had found the perfect place for Mom.

It had originally been established by the Dominican Sisters of Peace. The order's four guiding values in founding Lourdes were dignity, service, spirituality, and compassion. The order was dedicated to bringing the loving presence of Jesus Christ to people of all faith traditions or even none. It was simply the principle that guided their compassionate care. Although the nuns were still involved in the community, Lourdes was staffed by highly trained caregivers and medical professionals.

There was only one hitch. Lourdes was about to open a state-of-the-art memory care unit called Clausen Manor. Mom would be a member of the first class to take up residence there, so to speak. The rooms were small, individual suites with a bathroom, bed alcove, sitting area, and view of the grounds. There were community rooms, a spacious dining area, and activity centers. But none of it was yet ready for occupancy. That was the hitch.

So, Mom would live in a kind of communal setting called McFadden House until Clausen opened, a living situation that made her unhappy. She was passing through the late middle stage of Alzheimer's where she was still trying to deny and fight the disease. I think this is the most heartbreaking period for an Alzheimer's sufferer and her caregivers. As many families can tell you, there is a lot of anger, confusion, and fear.

continued on p. 196

• • •

I REMEMBER THE first story I published about Alzheimer's as editor-in-chief of *Guideposts*. It was by a daughter who was struggling with her widowed mother in that very belligerent stage of the disease (it must be noted that not every person with Alzheimer's goes through this stage).

To the surprise of some of my colleagues, I chose it as the cover, with a photo of Maria Massei-Rosato and her seventy-five-year-old mother, Josephine, of Brooklyn, New York. Josephine was holding a rosary and we just couldn't get a smile out of her.

Maria talked about the trial of going to her mother's house nightly and bathing her. Her mother would often turn caustic and abusive. "Get away from me," she'd scream, swatting Maria's hand. "I can do this myself!" Maria would remind herself of all the times in her life when her mother helped her when she didn't really want her to, even though she needed the help. It was a matter of pride and independence.

One afternoon when bringing her mom home from a doctor's appointment Maria asked her to wait while she bought a book. "Why are you doing this to me?" Josephine screamed in the middle of the bookstore. "You only care about yourself!" Five years earlier her mother never would have said anything like this, especially not in public. Customers and employees stared at the outburst. Maria paid for her book and hastened her still-angry mother out of the store.

That night she called a friend, Yvonne, in tears. Yvonne had experience caring for dementia patients. "Maria, I know it hurts you, especially coming from your own mother. You can't take it personally. Your mom's not really mad at you. She's frustrated that she can't do the things she used to do, even taking a bath. She's fighting. She's frightened. Just give her some space."

A few nights later Maria drove to her mom's house for the dreaded bath. She sat outside for a long time, staring at the familiar light glowing in the living room of the house where she had grown up. She remembered how her mom always left that light on for her so she would get home safe and sound, especially after her father died when she was ten. Her mother worked so hard to give her a good home. She prayed for the strength to help her mother now in her time of greatest need.

The light seemed like an answer to that prayer, a sign that God would guide her through these hard times. But she needed to understand that her mother was fighting against a terrible tide. Her mom was proud and independent and trying to hang on to the person she once was for as long as she could. It wouldn't go on forever. Until then, Maria would have to depend on her faith more than she ever had, to believe that the grace of God would light her way.

Maria's journey with her mother is one that countless caregivers will experience in the coming years as the population ages. With her story we published an

informational sidebar from the Alzheimer's Association
that is invaluable to anyone who is struggling to care for
a loved one with Alzheimer's (see the information
on p. 197–199).

S HORTLY AFTER MY MOTHER MOVED INTO McFADDEN HOUSE, I got
a call from Mary Lou.

"She got loose again," she said.

"Oh, no."

"This time a priest chased her down the road and brought her back."

"Don't tell me. She was trying to go home."

"That was the gist of it."

"This can't keep happening," I said.

"Someone probably left the alarm on the door off. They'll have to
be more careful."

My mother was proving to be a problem. And it wasn't just the
escapes. She had turned into a kleptomaniac of sorts. They found
items missing from other residents' rooms hidden among Mom's
things. This was totally out of character. Mom had never stolen anything in her life. She would rather die than take someone else's things.
The supervisor said the items Mom was swiping were not particularly
valuable: socks, candy bars, a pink T-shirt, and the like. They were
easy to retrieve and of course Mom claimed to have no idea how they
came into her possession, which was probably true. But we couldn't let
her go around lifting people's stuff in the night. That had to stop.

"The one item we had trouble finding was a little gold cross. She
had it hidden in her purse, and she really didn't want to give it back.
She tried to say it was hers."

A cross. Why would she steal a cross? Wouldn't that seem like sacrilege? A sin? No, I finally decided, this theft wasn't just random pilfering. It had meaning to her. She was trying to find something, to hold on to something. The cross was the ultimate symbol of her faith, and in that twilight that her mind was now inhabiting she knew it was the only thing she could take with her. She'd never talked much about what Cass and Marion—and her own father, for that matter—had gone through but it was surely something that she must have thought about. And now it was happening to her even as the awareness of what was actually happening dimmed. For her, that cross was not a stolen thing but the key to eternal life.

Still, she had to give it back. So, the next time I visited with her I brought her a little gold cross, which she put right into her purse, where all things valuable went.

Needless to say, we were anxious for Mom to be transferred from McFadden House to Clausen Manor on the Lourdes campus. We were confident that we had been led to the right facility for her but it couldn't come soon enough.

• • •

Choosing the right memory care facility is a complex challenge. AARP, The Alzheimer's Association, A Place for Mom, and Alzheimers.net among others offer comprehensive guidance for families seeking care for their loved ones. It is important to plan for your loved one's long-term needs as much in advance as possible.

Here are a few things to keep in mind as you're looking for the right facility for your loved one.

- **Location, Location, Location:** When possible, find a quality facility that can be easily visited by family and friends. If this isn't feasible, check if it has internet access, preferably broadband, so that you can use tools like Zoom and Facetime to keep in touch.

- **Staffing:** Some states have regulations governing the ratio of staff to patients so please check with the relevant agency. A 1:5 staff to patients ratio is generally considered optimal. An in-person visit will help you evaluate how staff interacts with residents. Ask what training is required for caregivers. Is there a nurse assigned to the facility? What are their hours? Does the facility have a medical director? Does it have a relationship with a doctor or hospital and provide dental services? Do they offer hospice care?

- **Activities:** Sing-alongs and music therapy, light exercise, puzzles, games, entertainment—all are beneficial to dementia patients. It is important that residents keep engaged with each other and their environment. Many facilities offer personal care such as hair styling and manicures.

- **Safety:** Investigate a facility's access points. Are they secure? Are there keypad entrances for family and staff? Does the facility offer emergency pendants and ID bracelets. Are they equipped with GPS chips? Ask about handrails and non-slip flooring as well as special night lighting in bathrooms, where falls are a risk. Bring a checklist of safety concerns to an in-person visit. Some state agencies keep a record of safety problems in nursing homes and memory care units.

- **Food:** Try to visit during mealtime and check out if the food is adequate and nutritious. Do they have a nutritionist on-site? Do they accommodate special dietary needs and allergies? Do the meals seem like something you would eat?

- **Faith resources:** Does the facility offer or have access to services and clergy? If not on-site, do they offer transportation? Faith remains central to many dementia patients even as other faculties erode. Their spiritual needs can be as important as their physical care.

CHAPTER TEN

MOM'S NEW BEST FRIEND

Eventually Clausen Manor was ready for occupancy and Joe, Toni, and Mary Lou moved Mom in, bringing along things from her house that would make her new surroundings more familiar: family photos, her "prayer works" suncatcher, a few small pieces of furniture, and the like. They bought a bed and a pretty quilt for it.

As soon as we could, Julee and I flew out to visit. Clausen really was state-of-the-art. It was bright and clean with attractive views and plenty of space. In my nightmares, I'd imagined that we'd someday have to warehouse Mom in one of those dreary, understaffed, decrepit nursing homes that are the fodder for undercover investigative reports on local news programs. Bedsores, overmedicating, and roaches in the food all breathlessly revealed by the intrepid reporter with perfect hair. "Imagine if your loved one landed here." Then a shot of several sketchy individuals handcuffed with their faces craned away from the cameras being frog-marched to a police van.

An old sponsor's words were once again proven true: "Our projections are always way worse than the reality."

We were greeted by a gracious nun, Sister Something-or-Other—I don't remember her name. That's a terrible thing for me to say since the early portion of my education was conducted by pious and dedicated nuns who made sure I paid attention. But I was anxious to meet the director of Clausen, Colleen Burke, about whom I had heard so many good things from Joe and Mary Lou particularly.

Colleen greeted us warmly and said, "I'll take you to Estelle. She's with her friend Pat."

Pat, I wondered, *Pat who?*

"Who's Pat?" Julee whispered.

I shrugged.

My mother was sitting at a table with another woman, presumably Pat. They'd just finished lunch. Had I not known what needs Clausen served, I would have thought these were just two seniors enjoying each other's company.

"Hi, Mom," I said. She rose to her feet, moving somewhat stiffly for her. I took note of that.

"You look great, Estelle!" Julee said, giving her a long hug.

Mom turned to Pat and said, after a moment, "Ed's girlfriend." She couldn't find Julee's name or the exact nature of our relationship. (Later, after we left, I lamented this fact to Julee. "She did the best she could," Julee said. "She knew I was someone you love.")

"Where did you come from?" Mom said to me, laughing with surprise, then turned to the other woman. "He's my youngest," she said.

"I've heard about you!" the woman said.

"My friend Pat. I told her everything," Mom said.

"You did?" I didn't know what to think about that, but I smiled anyway.

"It was quite a story," Pat said, nodding.

Mom was dressed casually but neatly, as always. Her sweater said, "Best Grandma," no doubt a gift from the girls. Pat was a bit more formal, dressed in a pressed peach pantsuit and clutching a purse that I later learned she never went anywhere without, even though it was permanently empty.

"We shopped at the mall," Pat said.

"That's where she got her outfit," Mom added.

Behind them Colleen was shaking her head no. They hadn't been anywhere.

"I tried to talk Estelle into getting one just like it, but she wouldn't. Maybe she's too cheap!" Pat said with a laugh.

"It's not my color, you should know that. In all these years, when have you known me to wear...that color?"

In all these years. Odd slip of the tongue. Clausen had only been open a month.

"Estelle, you wore that color at your wedding. I remember. It really showed off the red in your hair."

"I did?"

"Yes, I remember."

"I remember you being there. Maybe you wore that color."

"I probably did. But you did too, even when we were in high school. You drove all the boys crazy with that copper hair."

"You were just jealous," Mom said with a giggle.

"We liked the same boy, but Estelle got him!"

"You liked his brother, though."

"Yes, but the Sisters frowned on it. They were always after us about something!"

"Weren't they always," Mom said, nodding.

This conversation is getting surreal, I thought. Had they actually, inconceivably, known each other before Clausen? No one had mentioned this situation to me.

"Where are you from, Pat?" I asked.

"I'm from up in the thumb, I think." She paused. "Born and raised!"

Michigan is famously shaped like a mitten. The thumb is what we call the peninsula that juts out into Lake Huron. I used to camp on the beaches there in summer, counting the stars over the big lake and being eaten alive by sand flies.

"Pat, I think we're going to take my mom for a walk now. It's been nice meeting you."

"Thank you! Nice meeting you!"

I couldn't help noticing that Pat apparently took substantial advantage of the on-site salon, her thinning hair perfectly colored and coiffed, as opposed to Mom's thick, tousled gray hair. I have the exact same hair, though not yet fully gray, and inherited from Mom a certain indifference to styling it.

We headed to Mom's room so she could grab a sweater. She did a pretty good job navigating the hallways, with a little direction from an aide.

"This way, Estelle."

Outside her room was a little plaque with a picture of Mom as a beautiful twentysomething. I wondered if my dad had taken the shot. Probably. I wondered if she remembered who my dad was. I hoped so but couldn't bring myself to ask. He'd been dead for well over a decade.

While Julee helped Mom with a sweater they found in her closet, I took stock of the room. A small sitting area with a love seat, a reading chair, a bed, private bath. Mary Lou and Toni and the girls had done a wonderful job of adding little touches to make it feel homier. The bed was neat and squared away. The whole setup was a blessed relief. Mom would do well here.

"I like your room, Mom."

"Dad made the bed for me."

I didn't say anything. I knew better. Don't correct. Go with it.

"Mom made the quilt."

"It's gorgeous," Julee said.

• • •

So strange, the way the mind works. Even in her state Mom felt the need for the bed and quilt to have a story, even if it made no sense. That's what she and Pat did, merging their pasts to create a story of their lifelong friendship. Where their memories failed, their imaginations took over. It was a kind of confabulation taken to the next level and it was beautiful. Tapping into the power of their imaginations, they created new memories, as real in the moment as the ones they'd actually lived and lost. There was something inspiring in that, and comforting, the enduring yearning for story and the power of the imagination.

"I like your friend Pat," I said on our walk around the Lourdes campus, which Clausen was a part of.

"Did you know her son is a priest? Father, Father...Mike?"

I doubted this until I saw Pat sitting on a bench with a priest. We waved.

"He says Mass for us."

"Here?" I asked her.

"Yes, sometimes. He comes a lot." She smiled.

I tried not to let guilt get to me. Mom was doing so much better than I could have imagined. Joe, Mary Lou, and Toni had found just the right place for her. And this thing with Pat, their crazy lifelong friendship. What could be fundamentally lonelier than losing yourself? Now she had a friend and a past, of sorts, that served the purposes of the real past that was quickly falling away.

When it was time to say goodbye Mom said, "Come back anytime. It's not far." I promised we would.

· · ·

OVER THE NEXT FOUR YEARS I KEPT MY promise as often as I could, each visit making me more aware of my mother's inexorable decline, one I knew there was nothing to be done about. Facing the intractability of a disease is one of the most helpless and powerless feelings you can experience, which is why we turn so often, so desperately to prayer.

One time I surprised her in her room while she was saying the rosary. She didn't notice me come in at first, so I watched for a moment. I'd seen my mother say the rosary many times growing up. It was the most important part of her prayer practice. A rosary was always in reach. Now I watched her lips move and her fingers travel across the fifty-nine polished wooden beads of a rosary I'd found in Ecuador years before at a remote market high in the Andes just a few miles from the equator. I very clearly remembered buying it. One of my traveling companions, a glib Brit, said, "Once a Catholic always a Catholic," but another of my fellow travelers, Pip, a young nurse from New Zealand, leaned in and whispered, "She'll love it. You are a good son."

She still had it. She still remembered how to say it. Suddenly there was a lump in my throat. I found my lips moving silently with hers, "Our Father, who art in heaven…" Well, maybe not so silently. She looked up, confused. I'd startled her and for a moment it seemed like she couldn't place me. Then she smiled and I gave her a hug and she greeted me with her usual, "Where did you come from?"

Good question. From her, my father, their parents, and a lot of people I knew little about, all the way back to County Wexford, a Rube Goldberg confluence of genes through the generations. Who is it that can tell me who I am?

• • •

I VISITED MORE OFTEN AS HER CONDITION WORSENED. Her eyes always lit up when I arrived, and she usually was able to get up and hug me even though speech often eluded her. Frequently I'd find her sitting with Pat, Pat with her perpetual purse and immaculate clothing, talking about an imaginary past.

"The boys loved Estelle's bronze hair!"

I wondered how Pat could know the color of my mom's hair so many decades before they met. She seemed to know a lot about my mother that she couldn't have reasonably known, and I wondered how that could be, what strange interpersonal alchemy accounted for it. Or was it something more?

I was relieved, at least, that my mom had finally passed through the phase of the disease where she was battling it, that awful middle period where she knew what was happening but couldn't stop it no matter how hard she fought, like someone trying to outrun a landslide. She seemed to have reached a kind of equilibrium where she was at peace. I tried to think of that as a blessing while ignoring the erosion of her personhood, the entropy that was occurring in her neurons.

Every time I visited, she seemed to have faded a bit more, like an old photograph left out in the sun. She'd begun to shuffle more than walk. Still, I was able to take her out to lunch and carry on the semblance of a conversation. And she still complained about the allegedly excessive amount of food they served at the Olive Garden just down the road from Lourdes where I would take her. And maybe it was a learned behavior gained from years with my photographer-father, but she always smiled for the camera when I insisted on taking a picture, even if that smile was a little crooked these days.

One day I was sitting outside while Mom napped. Colleen Burke joined me.

"How's Green Eyes doing?" she asked, using her nickname for Mom.

"Doing as well as I can expect," I said. "There's a little less of her every time I come."

"Don't assume too much," Colleen said. "There's more there than you think."

"I worry she won't remember who I am."

"My experience is that on some level most people never really forget those they love. Maybe they lose the ability to express that recognition or form a thought around it, but deep inside I believe they still love."

"I guess you can't destroy love," I said, trying, I suspect, to convince myself of my thesis that love was indestructible, more metaphysical than just the process of neurons waltzing in the brain. I thought again how my mom's faith was still intact. It was hard to imagine that her love for her children could be erased even by something as devastating as Alzheimer's. I remembered what Julee said: "She knows I'm someone you love." Was love the one nexus of consciousness that endured the ravages of the disease? The one thing that still made sense? Or was my mother already gone, with only her body left to finish the last steps of her earthly journey?

"I love these people," Colleen told me. "That's why I stay here and do this work. The disease is sad, but so many of our residents are so loving."

Did Colleen see a cure or treatment on the horizon?

She shook her head. "We're still a long way off."

How long? A selfish little voice in the back of my mind asked.

• • •

BACK IN NEW YORK I FOCUSED ON MY work and my sobriety and talked to my twelve-step sponsor nearly every day.

"If sobriety is about anything it's about acceptance," he said over coffee one afternoon. "Acceptance of your alcoholism. Acceptance of your powerlessness. Acceptance of your higher power and His will for you."

"I have problems with that middle one."

"We all do, even civilians. As the Big Book says, who among us wishes to accept that we are powerless? We fight against it every day, even long after we no longer fight the urge to drink. But you just don't turn over half your will to God."

To this day I struggle with the concept, yet I know there is very little in my life that I am in complete control of. If you consider it, the accretion of a million factors plays into every minute of your life and the decisions you make…or don't make. Most of those million factors you have no control over, even though they determine the outcome of your decision.

There is a kind of quantum parlor game physicists play which postulates that there are virtually an infinite number of parallel universes where every decision or choice you did not make is still played out as if you did. I have no idea if this is true or why it should matter if it is, except theoretically. For me, though, it perfectly exemplifies the concept of powerlessness. We think we control so much when in truth we control so little. The smallest decisions we make, like a minor course correction for a large ship, can take us far in a different direction as time passes. Which is why, my sponsor explained, we surrender our will to God. Good. Orderly. Direction.

"You can't change the course of your mother's disease," he said, finishing his coffee and getting up. "You can pray for her, but you have to accept that there is nothing you can do to save her. And as to your own worries—which, by the way, are only natural and you should stop feeling guilty about them—you have no control over those either. You never know the future, only the probabilities. Wanting to know the future is wanting to be God. Don't do that."

These sessions always made me feel if not exactly good, then at least more focused.

• • •

ANOTHER THING I'D TAKEN TO DOING WAS LIGHTING candles at St. Francis. I've always liked lighting candles. As an altar boy, I lit the candles in the church before Mass and extinguished them when the service concluded. I loved the smell of candle smoke even though it aggravated my asthma.

It was the ritual of lighting a candle in the sanctuary at St. Francis rather than any meaning attached to it that attracted me, the remembrance of a long-ago duty. I wasn't even sure what it meant, only that my mother would probably appreciate me doing it for her. There was something mesmerizing about seeing the flame enlarge and illuminate the colored glass. I'd lapse into moth mode. One day a voice came up from behind me as I was staring into the flame.

"How is your mother?" It was Brother Barnabas.

"The same," I said, "And getting worse."

"It is the mind, right?"

"Yes."

"I have known it to happen to a number of our brothers in the order. It is a terrible thing to see, and I am sorry your mother and your family have to go through it."

"Me too."

"Remember, God is with you at all times, even when you doubt it, and I know, Edward, sometimes you doubt."

I said nothing in response.

"Doubt is as natural as belief, perhaps even more so. I don't think you can have faith without doubt. Sometimes we stress-test our faith."

"I feel I'm being tested constantly. It feels like I have already lost her."

"Perhaps you do feel as if you are being tested. But never forget that even in the throes of that feeling you are loved by God and are saved by that love. So is your mother. All He asks is that we love each other. All you can do now for your mother is to love her. Pray for her. Prayer is the greatest form of love, for yourself, for others, for God. With prayer, you are never powerless, and never alone."

continued on p. 212

• • •

A FEW YEARS back, *Guideposts* published a piece on what is called "ambiguous loss." It was a story from a woman whose husband's depression was so severe he had to be hospitalized in long-term care.

She experienced an intense grief even though he was still alive. Her sense of loss was as profound as if her husband had died. This is a phenomenon known to affect caregivers and loved ones of Alzheimer's sufferers in the final stages of the disease. One of our senior editors, Amy Wong, published a follow-up interview with an expert on the subject, social worker Susan Favaro, which I include here.

How to Cope with Ambiguous Loss

Unresolved grief is common for a caregiver of a loved one with dementia, depression, or another condition in which the person is present physically but changed or absent psychologically. There's a name for it—*ambiguous loss*, a term first used by family therapist Pauline Boss. Susan Favaro of the Banner Alzheimer's Institute talked about how caregivers can cope with ambiguous loss. Some tips:

- **Put a name to it.** Favaro believes the real culprit behind caregiver stress is the ambiguity of having a loved one who is lost only partially. "The grief of that leads to anxiety, ongoing strain, and confusion," she says. "It affects family relationships." Identifying this as ambiguous loss helps caregivers see "they're not crazy—it's the situation that's crazy."

- Use "both...and" thinking. Caregiving can involve holding two seemingly incompatible ideas at the same time. Instead of "either...or" extremes, try to think in terms of "both...and." Your loved one is not here or gone; he is both here and gone. You need to take care of both your mother and yourself. Think about how you would fill in the blanks: "Due to my caregiving experience, I have both lost [...] and gained [...]."

- Accept that good enough is good enough. "This is another Dr. Boss principle," Favaro says. "Doing things perfectly isn't possible with caregiving due to the uncertainty and unpredictability." Try to balance control with acceptance. Accept that you can't master the disease affecting your loved one, and take control of what you can: your thoughts, your reactions, tending to your own health.

- Manage your mixed emotions. Caregivers often have two conflicting emotions simultaneously. For example, thinking *I want this to be over* and feeling guilty because that means the person you're caring for would be gone. Guilt, anger, frustration—"it's normal to have these emotions, but we don't want to act them out," Favaro says. That's why it's important to share your feelings, and the losses and changes you experience, with others: friends, a support group, a pastor, a counselor.

- Imagine new hopes and dreams. "Think about what you can do to nourish yourself while you're providing care and what you'd like to do in the future," Favaro suggests. "Is there anything you can do now toward that? What would your family member want you to do in the future?"

I know now that I struggled with ambiguous loss in my mother's final months. Earlier in this book I compared her to a sailing vessel slowly disappearing into a fogbank never to be seen again. As her disease progressed, that fog became thicker and thicker to me. Yet even unseen, that vessel sailed.

THE LAST TIME I WAS WITH MY MOTHER was the spring of 1999, shortly after I had been named editor-in-chief of *Guideposts*, at the age of forty-six. (A reader who saw my picture with my first editor's note wrote to congratulate me, then added, "I hope you have some older people around to help you.") I knew how proud Mom would have been had she been able to understand. She would have been happy for my future. Visiting her, I believed she could sense my presence on some root level and that was enough. If she could have spoken, I'm sure she would have said, "Where did you come from?"

That spring I spent a week in Michigan house-sitting while Joe, Toni, and the girls took a much-delayed vacation in Florida. In the previous months, my mom had had several brief hospitalizations for urinary tract infections, a couple of falls, and other minor medical problems. My being there also gave Mary Lou a break while I spent time at Clausen. We were nearing the end and my siblings had been carrying so much of the weight.

But so had the staff at Clausen. When I first stepped into my mom's room, she was being attended to by people I didn't recognize. *Who are these strangers?* I wondered. *What are they doing here?* An aide dribbled sugar water through a dropper onto Mom's cracked lips, making rivulets of the deeper wrinkles on her chin. I noticed her friend Pat standing to the side, purse in hand. A woman was holding Mom's hand in hers. She turned and I recognized Colleen Burke. "Hey, Green Eyes," she said softly to my mother, "look who's here." Mom turned her head and made what I took to be an attempt at a smile. The effort must have been exhausting and it caused more sugar water to run down her chin.

The hospice nurse and social worker slipped in, and Mom's eyes brightened slightly even as she tried to fend off the hovering dropper. "Hi, Estelle," the nurse whispered.

For a moment I felt like an intruder. My mom had always been so fiercely devoted to her family. Yet here she was, dying, surrounded mostly by young strangers.

I made myself go forward. Colleen transferred Mom's hands to mine. Her grip was surprisingly strong, and she was pulling me closer even as she closed her eyes. I was exactly where I was supposed to be amid my mother's new family, the kind people who cared for her and loved her on a daily, hourly basis. Not strangers but helpers, angels in a way, there to ease her passing. In the coming days I would see how much they cared.

• • •

AS A TEEN, ST. JUDE WAS THE BANE of my existence. Not the saint himself, mind you, but a statue that repeatedly appeared in my room—compliments of my mother. Jude is known to Catholics as the patron saint of lost or hopeless causes.

His first appearances came when I was a severely asthmatic child and would often sit up half the night trying to catch my breath and trying just as hard not to call out for my mother. She was tired and had my brother Bobby to care for and I didn't want to disturb her. I would have taken all my potions and inhalers and an extra dose of a bronchodilator—one that also happened at that time to be a pill laced with phenobarbital since the active ingredient was a stimulant and in any case asthmatics were thought to be high-strung to begin with. Well, you'd be high strung too if you couldn't breathe. At any rate, I was unknowingly addicted to barbiturates at a very young age, which may explain some of the difficulties I had later in life and how my brain may have developed the way it did.

That's when Mom first put the statue of St. Jude on my dresser. I didn't quite know how I felt being categorized at age eight or so as a hopeless case. It was a bit unsettling. Still, the statue provided some comfort on those nights I sat on the edge of my bed wheezing, sometimes till dawn, my boyhood poodle, Pete, at my feet.

I never grew out of my asthma as our family doctor assured us that I would, but I improved and learned to live with it. By my teen years I was already beginning to drink and worse. I tightroped bad behavior with good grades and got away with a lot more than I had any right to. That's when Jude made a reappearance on my dresser. "What are you doing here?" I snapped and promptly exiled him to a hall closet. My mom was back to her old tricks.

A day or two later he reappeared. I found a sneakier place to hide him, but alas it was no use. He kept coming back. It became like a game we played. Where's Jude? I finally gave up, and Jude dwelled in my room until I left for college, though I turned his face to the wall and hung some anti-war beads on him.

After Mom moved into Clausen I was rummaging through some things in her house, since we would soon have to sell it, when I unearthed Jude from a bunch of junk of mine that Mom had saved. His right hand, which held up two fingers, had been amputated at some point, and a chip in his hair made him look like he was balding. His iconic green cloak was reasonably well-preserved. I smiled. I knew just what to do with him.

Now, as my mother lay dying, he occupied a spot on her nightstand as he once had mine, just a statue bought many years before at a religious gift shop. He was one of who knows how many others, thousands probably, not imbued with any powers in and of itself, but with a telling history between us of both hopelessness and hope.

"Remember that war we used to have over Jude?" I asked, not really expecting an answer. "Well, he's here in your room now. Checkmate."

• • •

I SLIPPED AN ICE CHIP BETWEEN HER LIPS and her eyes came open. Maybe she understood. I'd been spending these days mostly in her room, reading while she slept. Sometimes she would stir in her sleep, and I wondered if she dreamed. How do you dream without memories? Or are the deepest, most indelible ones set free in sleep?

All of the sadness I felt was momentarily swept away by a sense of gratitude. To be here sober, to be here when so many times I wasn't, to be here for someone who was always with me in prayer if not in person, whose love for me never faltered no matter how I tested it. Love that was as strong now as it ever was because that was all that was left.

I knew how unfair it was to unburden yourself to the dying, but I couldn't help myself. "I don't know how to say I'm sorry for all the terrible stuff I put you through, all the trouble I caused. I wasn't an easy kid, was I?"

The corners of her mouth seemed to turn ever so slightly into a smile. Or at least I wanted to believe so. I wanted to believe so much, in angels and grace and heaven and a life beyond this tangle of neurons and evaporation of memory, this seeming loss of self.

"I love you," I said. "I've always loved you no matter how I've acted. And I always knew you loved me even when I wouldn't love myself."

She raised her head slightly, slowly. Her lips moved and she said the last word I would ever hear her say, softly but clearly.

"Love."

. . .

I SPENT THE NEXT FEW DAYS SITTING IN her room, hardly noticing the comings and goings of aides and nurses. Sometimes I would look up and see Pat standing at the door.

I had coffee one afternoon with Colleen Burke. "How much longer?" I asked.

"Not too much, though some hold on longer than others. It's a process."

We'd declined the feeding tube, of course, and Mom had been diagnosed with heart failure, a common complication of Alzheimer's. I wondered if down deep she was fighting or simply letting go. Rossiters were fighters, Norman-Irish warriors. There was no way to tell. And yet my mom appeared to be at peace.

I left her on a sunny Saturday morning, giving her one last gentle hug. Joe, Toni, and the girls would be back the next day and Mary Lou was coming down that afternoon. I paused in the doorway to take one last look at the woman who had given birth to me. The room seemed incongruously bright. Her caregivers were attending to her. She was in good hands, God's hands. Then I turned and headed for the airport. On the way I stopped at a pay phone to call my sponsor.

"I feel so overwhelmed," I said.

"It's dying," he said. "We're supposed to feel overwhelmed."

. . .

ON MONDAY, APRIL 19, I WAS IN TUCSON, Arizona, helping teach a *Guideposts* writing workshop. Two senior editors were conducting the morning session. I would join them for lunch and the afternoon session then host a dinner that night.

Having once lived in Taos, I love the Southwest, and not just because it reminds me of my raw youth. There is a brute beauty to its landscapes, as if the farther west you go the more American America gets, in its newness and wildness. I might have stayed there forever if I could have found a way.

It was a crisp cool spring morning, and I was up early thanks to the time zone change. I wanted to hike Picacho Peak, but it would take hours I didn't have so I settled for the tamer and closer Tumamoc Hill near our hotel.

The path was easy for most of the hike but got steeper higher up and I was surprisingly breathless when I reached the top at a little over 3,000 feet. I lay on my back and looked up into the great western sky, a few tufts of clouds interrupting the boundless blue, a sky that seemed so vast yet so close. A spear of sunlight hit my eyes and I remembered that I had forgotten sunscreen and couldn't stay long like this. I thought of my mother's love of the sun and how it healed her.

And then I felt something, like a swooning of the soul, a gentle rush as if something were leaving, and at that moment I knew she was gone.

I hiked down quickly. There was a message for me at the hotel desk to call home. I knew already what the call would confirm.

There was no rush with arrangements since my mother was being cremated and Michigan weather could be iffy even in early spring, so we wanted to wait to give everyone time to attend her memorial service at St. Owen's. Then we would bring her ashes east later that summer for another small memorial and internment at Holy Cross Cemetery, where my father and Bobby were buried.

First, we requested an autopsy, which hadn't been done on Cass and Marion. We wanted to know for sure. The chief medical examiner at the time was the flamboyant and sometimes controversial Dr. Werner Spitz, who was an occasional adversary of my brother in court. Yet he generously performed the autopsy himself and confirmed that our mother had indeed suffered from and died of Alzheimer's dementia.

I have a recollection of seeing some of the images of tissue samples from her brain. Compared to a normal brain, one could easily detect the gaps and shocking shrinkage of gray matter. It was frightening, like something from a horror movie where a malevolent alien force attacks the brain. But in reality, it is the brain attacking itself. I thought of all the gaps where memories might have lived and breathed, where a sense of self was housed. But the soul? Looking at those images, at that labyrinth of brain matter, did not make me think of the soul, a soul that is improbably made up of neurons and glia. No, the soul is something more, something beyond that. It is a spiritual organ that transmits energy through us like a sacred current and cannot be destroyed, only freed. I'm reminded of an Emily Dickinson poem:

"The Brain—is wider than the sky—
    For—put them side by side—
    The one the other will contain
    With ease—and You—beside"

. . .

ON JULY 16 WE BROUGHT MOM HOME TO Philadelphia for burial. It was the very day that JFK Jr. died in a plane crash in fog over Martha's Vineyard. My mom admired the Kennedys. We were at Stone Harbor on the Jersey Shore when his father, John F. Kennedy, captured the Democratic nomination for the presidency in 1960. I remember Mom holding back tears. And later too when he won the presidency, the first Catholic, an Irish Catholic no less, to do so. My mother could still remember from her childhood the signs on businesses and rental properties that said, "No Irish need apply." Now one of her own was president.

She cried again watching little JFK Jr., known then as John-John, iconically saluting his father's casket after the assassination in 1963. I remember it too as something I would never forget, a dark and confusing moment to a nine-year-old that I knew would stay with me forever. And now it seemed that a circle had been closed somehow, in my mind at least.

CHAPTER ELEVEN

THINGS NOT FORGOTTEN

G ood morning, Dr. Salinas. Good to see you again."

"It's good to see you, Mr. Grinnan. Have a seat, please. How have you been?"

"Fighting off a chest cold but I'm at the tail end of it."

Walking to NYU Pearl I. Barlow Center for Memory Evaluation and Treatment on East 32nd Street on this April morning, one year after my first appointment with Dr. Salinas, I couldn't help marveling at how the city was transformed. It was now 2021, and the city almost resembled its former self, an old friend I recognized and wanted to hug. Some folks were still masked, even outdoors—we New Yorkers will not soon forget the devastating initial Covid-19 surge of March 2020—but the sidewalks roiled with people of all stripes, that wild diversity I love about New York. Cabs bleated through traffic. Pedestrians dodged bikes and vice versa. With the occasional admonition—ahem—given. The city looked like one big construction site with all the new buildings sprouting up. For years I've wondered where they will find the people to work and live in these glass and steel beanstalks, and year after year the people come. Now they were coming back.

Imprinted on my consciousness, as deep a memory crease as even September 11, is the night I fled New York in the teeth of the pandemic. We'd shut down the Guideposts offices in lower Manhattan. On that last day, one of the few remaining staff members discovered a couple old boxes of N95 masks left over from the anthrax scare in 2001 squirreled away in a storage closet. (At the time of the mysterious anthrax mailings, we had a particularly vigilant editor and part-time EMT who insisted that we not open mail without them. We may have rolled our eyes then, but we were counting our blessings now, literally.) We divvied up a box between us then donated the rest to a firehouse down the street. The young firefighter to whom we offered the masks seemed perplexed. But an older EMT snatched them and muttered, "We're going to need these."

"Technically, they're expired," I said.

"Technically, I don't give a damn," he replied.

That night, at what should have been crush hour, I boarded an Amtrak train at an eerily deserted Penn Station, headed for the Berkshires. I used my points to upgrade to business class—half a car at the rear of the train—thinking there would be more space between passengers and assuming the train would be jammed as usual. But there were only two of us in the car, a woman, masked, who sat in the first row, far right, and me, seated in the back row, far left, with my N95.

The geometry was unsettling. We could not have been intentionally farther apart in the car, and it felt strange to fear a fellow passenger, another human being, so entirely, and when she detrained two stops before me, I felt a shameful relief. Little did I know what was to come in the following months, and to this day I can't imagine losing the memory of that anxious exodus.

• • •

Dr. Salinas sat at the same sort of mobile desk unit where, as before, he took notes contemporaneously at the same typing speed I had previously envied. I was a little less fixated on his synesthesia this visit. Not afraid to scratch my nose for fear he'd mirror it.

He would publish his notes in my chart for me to read within hours, even minutes of our visit. I appreciate the openness of the process that gives you such immediate digital access to your health chart. There was a time when doctors wouldn't dream of letting you see your own chart even if you couldn't possibly read their handwriting. Well, perhaps I exaggerate but the transparency of the current process is surely striking. It's hard not to be aware of it as you converse with the doctor. NYU warns you that you may see test results before the doctor even reviews them. I can't imagine the consternation that might lead to given certain results.

We warmed up by reviewing the highlights of my last visit and the current state of my perceived memory issues. Recall that I was diagnosed with Subjective Cognitive Decline, a largely self-reported condition. I would like to take some narrative liberties in this section to include the doctor's notes, which I accessed immediately post-visit, that in retrospect now seems all a jumble.

DR's NOTES: *He is unaccompanied. He is alert, well-appearing, generally well, and is in his usual state of health. Appropriately interactive, cooperative, engaged. Calm, well-mannered. His affect is congruent, euthymic. "I feel good, slightly hyper."*

"Other than the cold, how are you feeling?"

"I feel good, slightly hyper."

I explained again that I had been at work on a book about Alzheimer's and my family, especially my mom's struggle, and my own fear of developing dementia and how it affects my view of the future. I had mentioned the project during our first appointment and said that I was now nearing completion of the manuscript and was largely satisfied with my work, though the medical and cognitive evaluation I hoped to explore had been slowed due to the pandemic, which frustrated me.

"I guess everyone is making up for lost time," I said. "It's impossible to get appointments." Immediately I regretted the comment, hoping he didn't think I was blaming him for the time it took to finally set up this visit. I didn't want to be taken as a complainer. That's the people-pleaser in me who comes out every now and again and probably not as often as some would like.

DR's NOTES: *Since his last visit he has been working on his third memoir which is about his risk of Alzheimer's disease. He feels his writing is as good as it has ever been, able to recall details of conversations and events in the past. When editing other manuscripts, he can remember if a previous edit of his, even at a granular level, has not been made and corrects it. Broadly speaking he feels his memory is good and he performs his professional duties ably. But describes "micro memory lapses," i.e., remembering events that happened sometimes only seconds before such as whether he applied the parking brake in his driveway or if he turned on the night light on his dog's collar. Endorses changes in memory. Endorses change in remembering details of recent events. Denies change in speech (though perhaps more difficulty in accessing certain words). Denies changes in language comprehension, handwriting, typing, or texting. Denies changes in behavior or personality. Denies that other people have commented on his cognitive functioning. Endorses history of alcoholic use disorder. Denies excessive guilt or hopelessness. Endorses history of excessive worrying.*

"As I said before, Doctor, it's as if that computer program that runs in the mind's background and performs tasks automatically without you even thinking about it is becoming glitchy."

Had my colleagues noticed anything about my memory?

No, not that they've said.

How about Julee?

Julee has frequently called me absent-minded, and occasionally declares I'm a genius for reasons that escape me because I'm most definitely not by any standards I've ever seen. But that is what a partner is for, I suppose. I shared this information with Dr. Salinas.

"But I've always been as smart as I needed to be," I added.

Dr. Salinas thought a moment, nodded, and made a note. I hoped I hadn't made myself sound ridiculous with this last comment, but it was true. My brain was like an engine that got me through life with a little extra in reserve when I really needed it. Was it that little extra that I felt possibly slipping away?

We moved on to the results of my MRI, which he said was unexceptional, as had my primary care doc when I showed him, though I still had some questions. I waited a moment while Dr. Salinas reviewed the findings.

DR's NOTES: *MRI brain (imaging) demonstrated mild small vessel degeneration and a right frontal parietal developmental venous anomaly, no clear evidence of atrophy or other intercranial abnormality.*

I don't know about you, but when words like *degeneration* and *anomaly* are mentioned in conjunction with a brain study, I squirm a little. Can you blame me? These terms, the doctor said, didn't imply anything serious or unusual and referred to changes in the brain typical of aging. They were, as my mother might have said, just doctor talk.

"So, my brain isn't perfect," I said, then remembered to smile. At least I didn't have any intercranial abnormality.

He nodded and made a note. I wondered if I had endorsed or denied something. (I understood these terms are not accusatory, merely professional idiom.)

We moved on to the memory tests, the part of the visit that made me nervous because last time I felt I had not performed well on some. We started by naming the months of the year backwards. I totally nailed it, though I restrained myself from doing a victory dance. There was one simple arithmetic test about making change, which I blew. *If you paid one dollar for three pencils at 28 cents each, how much change would you receive?*

"I was told there would be no math," I said, laughing.

I nailed the clock test as well, which entailed drawing the hands of a clock to indicate a given time, but that is the most basic test of all. If you fail that, you are in trouble.

Then came a series of word memorizations. This was where I had stumbled in my previous visit. The words were *face, velvet, church, daily, red, truck, banana, violin, desk, green*. I didn't think I had done any better this time and maybe worse. The more complicated the recall, the more lost and frustrated I felt, as if my memory was a house of mirrors. We finished up with some physical commands like touching my nose and pantomiming hammering a nail into a wall, all of which I could have done in my sleep. I was far more concerned with how I performed on word memorization and recall. Frankly, my recall sucked.

DR's NOTES: *Functionally Mr. Grinnan is at the level of subjective cognitive decline bordering on mild cognitive impairment compared to prior level of performance with amnestic pattern. Presentation is most likely multifactorial in etiology (e.g., sleep disturbance, possible component of rumination or mood symptoms, possible attentional change related to respiratory tract infection). However, the possibility of neurodegenerative disease such as Alzheimer's remains. Provided counseling and education today on his current risk factors (including discussion regarding his family history) and protective factors (including his highest level of education). At this time, he would benefit from further diagnostic characterization.*

"I would like you to see a neuropsychologist for further testing and evaluation, which I think would be helpful."

I nodded, realizing that my sense that I had done worse this time on some of the memory tests was confirmed. He also mentioned the possibility of an evaluation of my sleep patterns and habits, as I told him I usually get by on six or six-and-a-half hours most nights, which has always been the norm for me. I'm not sure I can sleep more than seven hours. Besides, I'd gone to bed preemptively early the night before this visit and it didn't seem to help me on the tests. Dr. Salinas typed out a few more notes as I gathered my things and took my leave.

"Thank you, Doctor."

"You're welcome," he replied softly, not looking up from his notes, notes I would soon be reading the minute they were uploaded to my chart. I stopped in the lobby to consult with his assistant. "Unfortunately, Mr. Grinnan, our neuropsychologist is booked through the year [this was April, mind you]. I can get you on her schedule in early January and put you on a cancellation list. Meanwhile, here's a list of some other neuropsychologists who might be able to see you sooner. Good luck and you'll hear from me if something opens up."

• • •

I LEFT WITH THE LIST AND HEADED TOWARD the East River Esplanade to find a place to sit and think. I don't really regard the East River as a river, more like a tidal canal connecting Upper New York Bay with the Long Island Sound, all of sixteen miles of heavily dredged waterway. It pales in comparison to the Hudson, a real river.

Still, it's the bridges that give the East River its personality, among them the Brooklyn Bridge, that monumental feat of 19th-century engineering and John Roebling's Teutonic will; its humbler sibling, the Manhattan Bridge, just upriver, in the shadow of which the Guideposts softball team used to play its games; the Williamsburg Bridge, which was once the artery for immigrants fleeing the teeming tenements of Manhattan's Lower East Side for the greener pastures of Brooklyn; the Queensboro Bridge, which most New Yorkers call the 59th Street Bridge recently renamed for ex-mayor Ed Koch but should probably be named after Paul Simon who wrote a hit song about it and didn't call it the Queensboro Bridge. There's the Rikers Island Bridge, which I never want to cross.

I walked toward downtown when I hit the esplanade and found a bench at Stuyvesant Cove. I watched some of the river traffic, mostly tugs and barges, and checked my phone. There was a message from Julee. "How did it go?" I figured I should look at my clinic notes and see.

"He is unaccompanied…"

I read through Dr. Salinas's observations. I saw my scores on the memory tests and noted they were a couple points down from the first visit…eight out of ten last year, six out of ten this year and so on, with more perseveration. I read his possible explanation for that decline. Then I saw the phrase "subjective cognitive decline bordering on mild cognitive impairment." Then the kicker: "The possibility of neurodegenerative disease such as Alzheimer's remains."

I was tempted to fling my phone into the river. I even wondered if I could make it skip. I wasn't angry. At least I couldn't tell if I was angry. I just felt like I should do something. Some pointed gesture. To react somehow to this diagnostic penumbra I was wandering through. I tried to mentally get my balance back. "Bordering on…the possibility of…."

• • •

EARLY IN THIS BOOK I ASKED MYSELF, IF I could know, would I want to know? Now I wondered if I could accept half an answer. Was that worse than knowing? At that moment, staring across the East River into Brooklyn, it felt like it was.

In some ways a diagnosis is a way to see into the future if the course of the disease is well understood, especially a disease like Alzheimer's that is largely untreatable and fatal usually within eight to ten years. Many patients die earlier, often from the complications of other conditions or just because they are lucky. My mother and her sisters were all healthy, so they played out the string.

Lord, what am I to make of this information? Is this your way of reminding me that nothing about my future is certain except You? That faith trumps knowing?

As I sat and pondered my predicament, I thought I might follow through with the neuropsychologist. Perhaps I could get some answers about my alcoholism and head injuries. It still felt like my history might have given the disease a head start, so to speak. How many brain cells had I squandered?

An elderly couple made their way toward the bench next to mine, the woman helping the man sit down. When she got him settled, she pulled two bottles of water from her bag, handed one to the man and sat down.

"What is this for?" the man asked, staring at the bottle.

"It's water, hon," she said.

"I don't drink water. I never drank water..."

The woman untied her head scarf and tucked it in her coat at the throat. "You'll need it when you get thirsty. You'll thank me." Then she buttoned the top button of the man's coat. "Gets chilly here by the water."

"The water?"

"The river, see? That's a barge or something."

"Are we going to a…baseball game?"

"No, not today, love."

The man started to open his water bottle, holding it sideways. The woman took it from him and opened it herself and put it in his hands upright. I'd seen this act before…the husband and wife in HoJo's when I was a busboy. These two were surely wife and husband as well. Their interactions bespoke so much fluid familiarity and casual tenderness.

Funny how a person with Alzheimer's tries to piece his world together even as it is falling to pieces. Not far from us was the East River ferry terminal. One place you could take a ferry to was the ballpark. Had this man done that in his past? Was he an unfortunate Mets fan? I wondered what she was thinking. About a future where she could no longer take him for walks along the water? Or did she live in the moment with her husband, in the diminishing margins of his life, where she could still love him the most?

The woman noticed I was staring at them. Not staring but taking note. Still, she noticed and gave me a smile. That smile. It came almost from another world, their world, the singular, sorrowful journey they were on, the journey I wanted to know if I was starting. Or did I?

I smelled the diesel fumes from a passing tug. It tooted its baritone horn. It was time to go.

• • •

AFTER ATTENDING TO A FEW ERRANDS AND STOPPING back at our apartment to grab my bags and a few things Julee claimed she couldn't live without, I was able to catch an earlier train than I had planned. I was back on an Amtrak with a good window seat to watch the sun dip below the Palisades. I stared out over the Hudson for a long time, watching the shadows darken the water, the ripples of a fish swimming close to the surface near shore. I tried to read yet another book on brain health but couldn't stick with it. I switched to an Irish thriller I'd started on my last trip to the city and finished it before my destination of Hudson, New York.

Nearing my station, we passed beneath the Rip Van Winkle Bridge, its name compliments of Washington Irving. I'd recently read of a young woman who jumped to her death from the span. The water must have been very cold.

Is suicide ever morally or religiously justifiable? Do you have the right to end your life while it's still a life? I can imagine that the woman who jumped off that bridge was probably trapped in a moment of extreme despair and hopelessness. She could not see a future free of unbearable suffering. Yet she did have a future, at least in terms of the actuarial charts. It was obscured by the pain she felt in that dark moment. She just wasn't willing to give life any more chances. She saw no other way out of her pain. I am almost certain she lost any sense of God in her life or a connection to the divine. Without God or hope, what was left to live for?

But what about someone who is nearing the end of their life with an intractable disease robbing them of it bit by bit, day by day? Does that person have the right to end their life before the disease inevitably and cruelly does? Especially a disease like Alzheimer's that removes the knowledge of who you are or even if you are alive. If you know for sure that that is your future, can you decide to take your own life before the disease renders you incapable of making that choice? Does our faith allow us that choice?

Jesus went to His death willingly, knowingly. He understood his fate with absolute certainty before His ministry on Earth began. Was His life a suicide mission? It's pointless and even blasphemous to call Jesus's crucifixion suicide when He could reclaim life and rise from the dead. Yet isn't that the promise of Jesus's death and resurrection? That we will overcome death with life everlasting? Death as an interruption rather than a full stop?

I don't mean to trouble you with these questions but increasingly people are asking them, especially with respect to fatal neurodegenerative diseases that strike late in life. I can't imagine ending my own life, and I am sure my mother never contemplated ending hers even after watching her closest loved ones and their families endure the agonies of Alzheimer's. Maybe it was her faith that made suicide unthinkable. Maybe it was denial. I imagine it was a bit of both plus the human will to fight for survival until the very end. But can I say with confidence that others who regard suicide as a morally and religiously viable option are defying God's will?

I don't have the answers, but I certainly do have the questions and I don't think it would be honest not to ask them, particularly in this context. It's different than leaping off a bridge before life has offered you a chance at redemption. I'm not sure if that woman asked for forgiveness before she jumped; I am not sure she had to. There is a difference, I suppose, between murdering yourself and euthanizing yourself with a clear conscience. I just don't know if we can ever figure out for sure where that line is or if it is right to decide it for others.

My train pulled into Hudson a little after dark. There was a cab there waiting for me. It was easier than having Julee drive over and pick me up then have to drive back. Besides, Amanda, the driver, is a friend. Times are tough for local cab companies. We liked helping keep her in business. Also, Amanda is an inspiration. She has gone through so much medical pain and suffering that she should change her name to Job. And still, in her mid-forties, she does not abandon hope.

"How's it going?" I asked, throwing my bag in back.

"The same. I can't complain. I mean I could, but I won't."

"I don't mind."

Amanda rattled off a list of tests she'd undergone that week and the hours driving back and forth to doctors and arranging more appointments. I think she was glad to get that information out of her system. I didn't say much. I didn't need to.

Eventually we fell to discussing our dogs and new hiking trails we'd discovered in the Berkshires. This one is unmarked. That one is not maintained but has fabulous views. We talked about bear sightings and our respective encounters. With sunset behind us, the old hills rose out of the Hudson Valley, gray-green in the distance. I thought about how they were once great high peaks, jagged and snow-capped, now smoothed over by time and geology, gentle rises in the earth, full of trails both marked and unmarked, and unforgettable views that will never be forgotten.

CHAPTER TWELVE

LOVE IS WHAT SURVIVES

The other day I found myself staring at a picture on my phone of a movie star, one whose talents I admire. I've seen many of his movies since the time I was in middle school. Yet now I could not for the life of me recall his name. It was somewhere in my brain, but I could not dislodge it. And people think of me as a movie maven.

I knew and liked this actor so much that I would watch a movie simply because he was in it. I could recall many of his great roles, hear his resonant voice and intonation, but I could not retrieve his name no matter how I tried. This was crazy! How could I forget such a famous name? I did not want to give in to Google. I forced myself to try and remember.

Still, the name did not come. I was getting a headache when I surrendered to Google and put in the title of one of his movies. The name appeared at the top of the credits. I felt a surge of recognition: Donald Sutherland.

How could I forget Donald Sutherland? He's appeared in nearly 200 movies, to say nothing of his commercial voiceovers, with his distinctive Canadian accent. I asked myself again was something wrong with me. Any number of my friends say forgetting stuff is normal as we age.

Still, these little slips of the mind trouble me. I have what I described to Dr. Salinas as lapses in micro-memory, events or actions that happened only minutes before. I apply the parking brake of our jeep at the top of our driveway and kill the engine. In that brief interval I become uncertain that I applied the parking brake. I doubt my memory. My brother says that sounds more like OCD than memory loss. But these little micro-memory slips pile up over the course of the day…except when I remember to remember. If I remind myself to remember something I usually remember it. It just takes that extra step. Am I compensating or just being practical? Why didn't I have to do this five years ago?

· · ·

I'M ENROLLED IN SEVERAL ONLINE BRAIN HEALTH PROGRAMS that involve testing. I like tests and games and puzzles. Yet there is one in particular I struggle with—pattern recognition. In short, you are shown a selection of patterns. In the next screen you are shown more patterns in addition to the patterns already shown, this time in different positions. You are asked to identify the previous patterns and their previous positions. Or something like that. See? I can't quite remember the rules.

At any rate my performance has apparently declined over the past year, where you would think it might improve with practice. At the conclusion of the test, I am invariably asked if I experienced distraction during the test (yes, Gracie was barking at the deer in our yard). How bad was the distraction? Was it worse than the last time you took the test? Do you think it impacted your score?

Are other people typically asked these questions or did my performance trigger the inquest?

I'm no fool. I know what they're getting at. I suck at this test and I'm getting worse. That's the pattern I recognize. But does it really mean anything? How does it apply to real life?

I think of human memory as primarily pictorial (as opposed to Gracie, whose memory is primarily olfactive—she has 300 million olfactory receptors in her nose to my meager six million; she smells the deer before she sees them). In this concept of memory, the mind is continually taking pictures at a rate nearing the speed of light; all that we perceive visually is actually pictures of the past, given the speed of light and the time it takes to reach the eye. Think of the sound effect your iPhone produces when you snap a picture, then multiply it nearly to infinity. That's how fast our brains are running. In fact, the brain indulges in visual editing. For instance, our noses are within our line of sight. Close one eye and we can see it. Or simply focus on your nose and it shows up. Normally we don't notice our nose even though it is there in our visual field. The brain simply edits that information out. Thanks, brain. But what else are you editing out?

We organize these pictures virtually instantaneously into our perceptions of reality and our thoughts. It happens so quickly, so automatically, that we are unaware of the process. Yet it is all based on those pictures, which are pictures of the past. All pictures are memories, and it is memory, therefore, that really forms our perceptions of the immediate present. The brain then stores and uses these memories to help construct our past. Or as the Italian theoretical physicist Carlo Rovelli observes in his book *The Order of Time*, memories hold together our sense of identity.

The foregoing is my simplification of several theories of the mind. But all emphasize the incredible role our memory function provides in shaping our thinking and decision making without us even being aware of it. Memory isn't just how we remember the past. In good measure it's how we experience the present, which is why my micro-memory fails trouble me.

You can well imagine then how the gradual derailment of these complex functions eventually render life unlivable without intense and constant caregiving, first by family members and then by professionals in nursing homes and memory care facilities.

• • •

B UT LET'S RETURN TO THE QUESTION I ASKED at the beginning of this book: Where does it begin?

I'm reminded again of the word Greek philosophers used to signify when a character recognizes his true nature or the true nature of a dilemma or the true nature of another person or dilemma: *anagnorisis*— the conversion of ignorance to knowledge.

Most families experience such a moment of Alzheimer's anagnorisis, though the path from ignorance to knowledge can wind through a baffle of denial. Still there comes a time when we arrive at the inevitable and painful conclusion that a loved one's mind is under assault. We can no longer write the behavior off to the vagaries of aging.

If you and your family struggled with denial before you finally came to terms with a loved one's true dilemma—Alzheimer's—you are not alone. Most families, including mine, resisted that realization. It is only human to do so. Be kind to yourself in this regard. But what if it is your own state of mind that you recognize as failing?

I began by telling you about the winter night I forgot to turn on Gracie's collar light and the ensuing questions it prompted. This morning I forgot to put her collar on altogether when I let her out. I should have finished my coffee first but instead I found myself trying to wrangle Gracie in my robe and bare feet as the sun peeked over the hills. Fortunately, the prospect of breakfast was more immediately appealing to her than the chance to charge through the underground fence with impunity.

I started this story by positing that wanting to know is a fundamental human desire. Wanting to know the future, wanting to know our fate, wanting to know God's will. That wanting to know, I wrote, was central to my quest to understand my own susceptibility to a dementia that runs in my family. Do I still want to know? Do I want to know how the story could end?

The backdrop to this book was the upheaval of the Covid-19 pandemic, which brought death to our collective front door as never before. As I was finishing the manuscript I lost my wife, Julee, who suffered from lupus erythematosus. Her lifelong struggle with a disease that brought her to the brink of despair was heartbreaking. For a time, I wasn't sure I would finish this work. It was Julee who urged me to embark on this journey even though she feared what I might find out.

On a practical level the pandemic disrupted and delayed medical appointments and tests. As I write this, I'm still waiting to undergo the further testing Dr. Salinas recommended, tests that will delve further into my cognitive issues. The appointment for this testing is still two months away, which gives me pause to consider if I am still willing to undergo the process, which will yield a more definitive diagnosis. I think about Dr. Salinas's observation that Alzheimer's remains an open question each time my memory falters.

Do I still want to know? In a way I've brought on this dilemma myself by asking. I've sought answers I believed I needed to know. I thought knowledge was power. But power over what?

That is a question I still can't resolve. Certainly, a finding of early cognitive decline gives one a chance to treat it with lifestyle changes, mental exercises, even experimental treatments.

Yet there is no power greater than love, the love of family, of friends and colleagues, and most of all the love of God, the most protective factor of all. It was my mother's last word to me for a reason. It's what I am convinced survives even the ravages of dementia, a love that can touch us even from heaven.

• • •

THERE IS A MEMORY I HAVE THAT I hope will never leave me. Back on the first anniversary of my mother's death, I awoke to a wet and blustery Saturday in the Berkshires, the kind of raw April day that makes spring seem like a broken promise. I'd planned a hike to a favorite lookout in Beartown State Forest, a remote trail that was finally open after an exceptionally rude winter. The weather had sabotaged my plans and I found myself wandering aimlessly through one of the musty secondhand bookstores for which this part of Massachusetts is known.

I needed another book like I needed a hole in my head, as Mom would have put it. I missed Mom saying things like that, missed them more than I ever imagined I would. I thought her long decline had prepared me for her death, but it was those little things more than her absence from this world that sometimes stirred up unexpectedly poignant moments. For an instant I flashed on Pat, standing in her pressed pantsuit with an empty purse. I wondered what had become of her after Mom died, though I knew what eventually would.

As my eye roamed the unkempt shelves, the title on a worn red spine jumped out at me: *The Southpaw's Secret*.

It was a boy's book, part of a short-lived Mel Martin mystery series by John R. Cooper that I'd been crazy about when I was a kid. Mel Martin was a high school baseball star and a wily young sleuth to boot. The books had already gone out of print by the time I read the two volumes I'd inherited from my brother, but I was hooked. I don't know how many hours Mom spent helping me hunt down the other Mel Martin books.

Mom was an intrepid sleuth herself, especially when it came to finding obscure things for me that I absolutely had to have. A rare Beatles album, for instance, which came out right before *Meet the Beatles!* was released and the band appeared on *The Ed Sullivan Show*, changing the course of the decade single-handedly. The elusive LP had the same songs yet with a different cover and I absolutely had to possess it. Mom somehow discovered the last remaining one at a small electronics store in Walled Lake, Michigan, about thirty miles from our house, and she drove there to get it before anyone snatched it up. Then there were the pair of used Cooper goalie pads I needed since I couldn't afford new ones. Mom spent half her time finding obscure stuff I had to have.

Except for *The Southpaw's Secret*, the one Mel Martin book she was never able to track down. And now it had found me after all these years on this rainy April day. Oh, and I did I tell you? My mother was a natural lefty.

• • •

A COLD NOSE NUDGES ME. GRACIE, REMINDING ME it is past time for a hike in the woods. We'll find a trail that will take us to a hilltop where we will sit and catch our breath and allow the view to lift us higher, where the wind sways the tops of the trees below. She'll sniff the breeze while I gulp some water. The lesson I have learned most in writing this book is the power of the present, of being present. The future is a black box. The now is where our faith intersects with our lives, where each day is another step on that journey of faith.

Acknowledgments

THE CHALLENGE OF ACKNOWLEDGEMENTS, AT LEAST FOR THIS author, is where to begin and where, finally, to end. When I think of all the people who have helped and loved me along the way, and without whom this book would never have been written, the list is indeed never-ending.

Still, what author can hope to succeed without a great—and patient—editor? I had two, Beth Adams and Carolyn Mandarano. As always, I am deeply indebted to Amy Wong who knows my writing, blemishes and all, better than anyone, and Colleen Hughes for reading an early draft and whose encouragement was indispensable.

Many thanks to John Temple, Dave Teitler, Kelly Mangold, Ansley Roan, Jimmy Lee, and the senior staff of Guideposts for giving me the time and space to complete this book, as well as Margaret Peale Everett, Elizabeth Peale Allen, Katie Berlandi, Wilma Jordan, and the Guideposts board of trustees.

If you have gotten to this page, you know that nothing could have preceded it without the help (and memories) of my brother, Joe Grinnan, my sister, Mary Lou Dillon, and my sister-in-law, Toni Grinnan. Thanks to my cousin, Carol Ambacher, and Colleen Burke, director of Clausen Manor, for kindly sharing their recollections of my mother and her journey. And to Rick Hamlin for his faith and friendship.

Much appreciation goes to Guideposts creative director Kayo der Sarkissian, photo editor Kevin Eans, book designer Pam Walker for the excellent cover and interior, and photographer Amy Etra. An additional tip of the hat to researcher Jaylin Rumph, copy editor Kirsten Anderson, Celia Gibbons, Celeste McCauley, Lu Broas, Bill McGlynn, Julian Lama, Jamie Anastasio, Chris Mellor, Jim Hinch, Roberta Messner, Rocco Martino, Laura Ross, Doc Emrick, Rosie Schaap, David Matt, Amanda

Kramer, and Michelle Amstead. Special thanks to Evelyn Freed for her steadfast friendship.

This book began in the early, frightening days of the pandemic when my wife, Julee, and our golden retriever, Gracie, fled Manhattan for our vacation home in the Berkshires of western Massachusetts. Julee died there in the spring of 2022—of health complications not related to Covid—and I only wish she could have been here to see this book to its completion, share in the satisfaction, and accept all the gratitude and praise she deserved. I pray that gratitude reaches heaven.

Ultimately gratitude is a gift to oneself. Voltaire said it best: "Appreciation is a wonderful thing. It makes what is excellent in others belong to us as well."

A Note from the Editors

We hope you enjoyed *A Journey of Faith,* published by Guideposts. For over 75 years, Guideposts, a nonprofit organization, has been driven by a vision of a world filled with hope. We aspire to be the voice of a trusted friend, a friend who makes you feel more hopeful and connected.

By making a purchase from Guideposts, you join our community in touching millions of lives, inspiring them to believe that all things are possible through faith, hope, and prayer. Your continued support allows us to provide uplifting resources to those in need. Whether through our communities, websites, apps, or publications, we inspire our audiences, bring them together, and comfort, uplift, entertain, and guide them. Visit us at guideposts.org to learn more.

We would love to hear from you. Write us at Guideposts, P.O. Box 5815, Harlan, Iowa 51593 or call us at (800) 932-2145. Did you love *A Journey of Faith*? Leave a review for this product on guideposts.org/shop. Your feedback helps others in our community find relevant products.

Find inspiration, find faith, find Guideposts.

Shop our best sellers and favorites at
guideposts.org/shop
Or scan the QR code to go directly to our Shop